G000074978

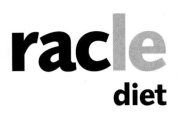

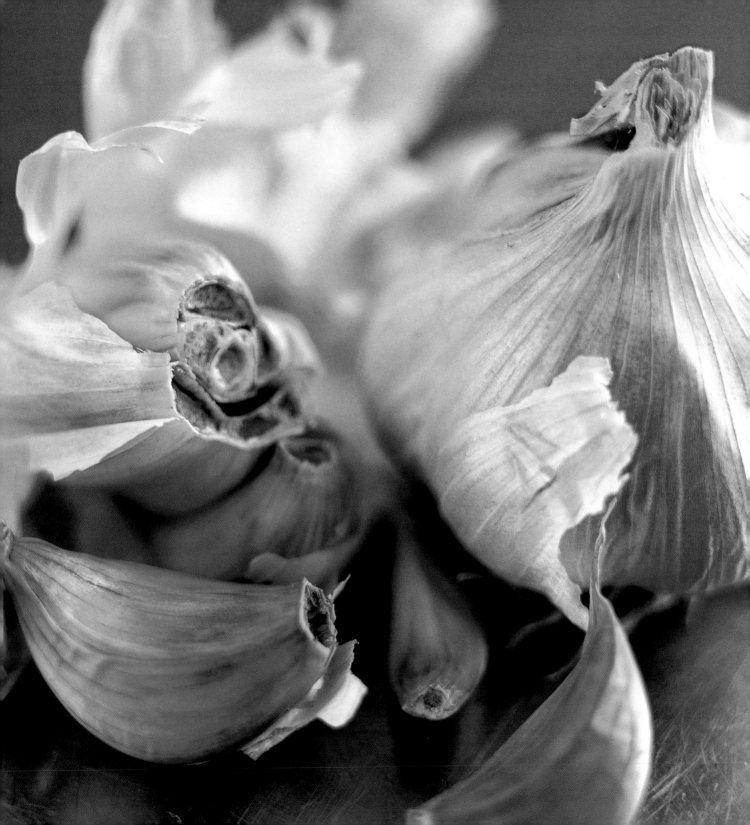

THE
oracle
diet

MICHAEL VAN STRATEN

Recipes by Sally Pearce and Michael van Straten

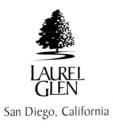

LAUREL
GLEN

San Diego, California

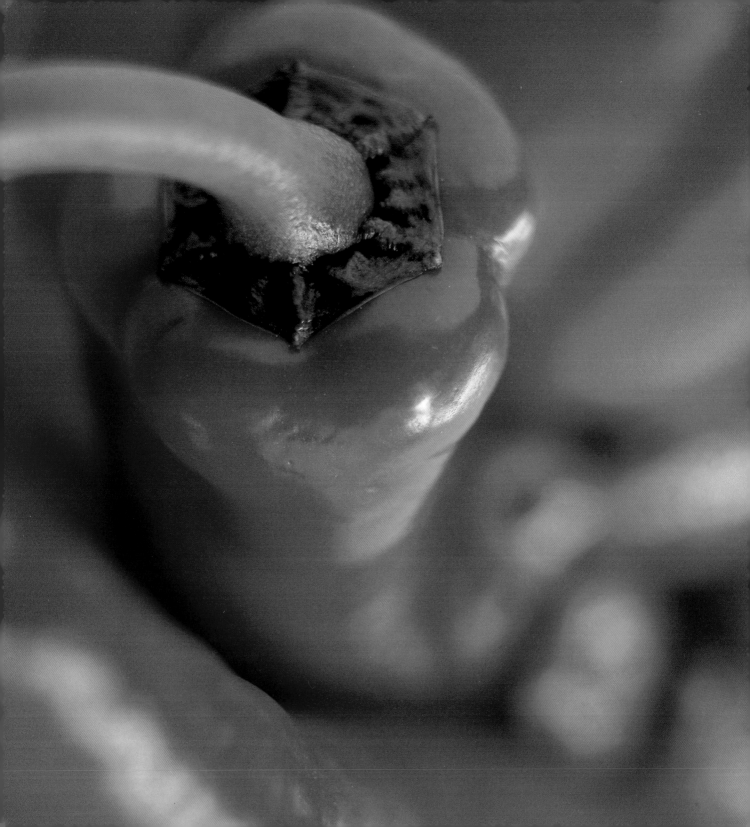

contents

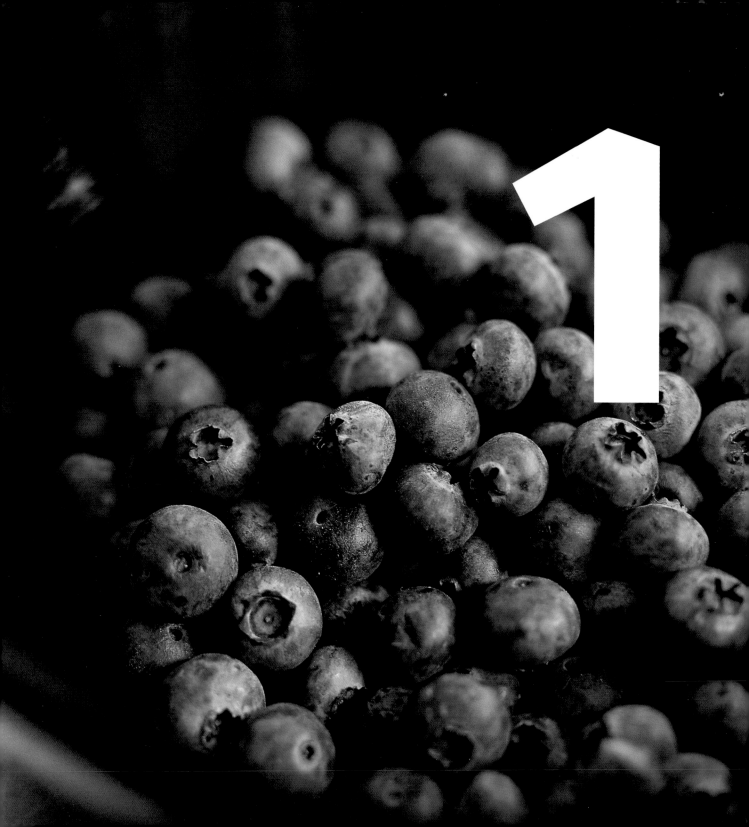

When the ancient Greeks needed answers to the most difficult questions, they went to the temple at Delphi to consult the oracle of the god Apollo. When the questions were really complicated, the supplicant was given an herbal drink to promote deep sleep and dreams, and spent the night in the temple. During these dreams Apollo appeared to the supplicant and handed down the oracle, and often cured medical problems at the same time.

introduction

Another famous oracle was at the temple of Asclepius at Epidaurus, the site of the very first hospital and the place where Asclepius perfected some of the earliest forms of surgery.

With these ancient health connections, there couldn't be a more appropriate word than "oracle" to describe the diet that you'll find in the following pages. And before you even think of counting calories, or of weight loss or starvation plans, I must tell you that they have no place here.

The ORACle Diet is unique among modern health and food books. It's about eating and enjoying delicious meals. It's about optimal nutrition and minimal fuss. It's about maximum benefit and the least possible damage to your body. It's about pleasure, not guilt.

The way we eat has changed more in the last 100 years than in the previous 100,000—and I've watched in horror how these changes have accelerated during the forty years since I first became involved in alternative medicine. As a naturopath, I use nutrition as the platform on which all health is based. Without good food, there can never be good health. But changing lifestyles, lack of skills in the kitchen, increasing time pressures, and the determined efforts of the food manufacturing industry have pushed us into a vortex of ever-decreasing nutritional value and ever-increasing consumption of health-damaging foods.

There's no doubt that freezers, microwaves, and instant meals have brought convenience to everyday living. But at what price? In spite of ever-increasing affluence, dramatic advances in medicine, and the ability of surgeons to replace most parts of the body with donor organs or artificial implants, health in the Western world is in steep decline. It's true that we've conquered smallpox and the plague. And there are vaccines to protect children and adults from many communicable diseases, drugs that control blood pressure and diabetes, scanners to detect the tiniest changes deep within the body, and ever more successful treatments for many types of cancer.

Nonetheless, we have major health problems. Heart disease is the number one killer in the United States: Cardiovascular diseases are responsible for 41 percent of all deaths. Sperm counts have decreased by 50 percent in the last fifty years, and infertility problems have soared. Nearly two-thirds of our adult population and an increasing number of children are obese. Allergies such as asthma, eczema, and hay fever are ten times more common than they were thirty years ago. And when life expectancy is increasing and more people are retiring early, these golden years are plagued by diabetes, arthritis, poor eyesight, osteoporosis, and Alzheimer's disease.

You may find it hard to believe, but your food—and the food you give your children—holds the key to the prevention or reduced risk or impact of most of these problems. Scientists have known for decades that essential vitamins, minerals, and trace elements play a vital role in both the preservation of life and the maintenance of good health, but it's only in recent years that the overwhelming importance of antioxidants has been acknowledged. It's these protective chemicals that fight against the damaging free radicals that attack cells throughout the body.

The ORACle diet is not only a delicious way of eating: it provides a natural path to health and vitality, dramatically increases your chances of disease-free progression into maturity, and is the simplest possible way of adding years to your life and life to your years.

It's time to stop worrying and love your food

Helena Rubenstein, the great pioneer of the cosmetics industry, said you should never put anything on your face that you wouldn't put in your mouth, and how right she was. No amount of expensive lotions and potions will help stave off the relentless march of time and aging unless you're eating the right foods. And the key antiaging foods are fruits and vegetables.

Medical science has conquered the ravages of most infectious diseases, surgeons can give you a new heart or a new hip, drugs can keep you mobile as the joints begin to stiffen, sewage systems and safe drinking water have eradicated killer epidemics of dysentery and typhoid in the Western world, but all this is papering over the cracks. Aging is a relentless march of nutritional deficiencies, and in spite of worldwide population studies and major research in the most prestigious university laboratories, the medical profession in general ignores the relevance of nutrition and its antiaging function.

It's simple: Every one of you can slow down and even reverse many of the body's natural aging processes, and you'll not only feel better and look better, but you'll gain enormous protection against the scourges of heart disease and some cancers. All you have to do is eat more of the very specific foods that are richest in nature's defensive chemicals—the antioxidants.

Fighting free radicals

Oxidation is a damaging process caused by a group of chemicals called free radicals, which are produced mainly when the body burns up the oxygen we breathe to keep us alive. We're also subject to damaging free radicals that get into our system from the outside as a result of smoking, environmental pollution, radiation, too much sunlight, and irritant chemicals that make contact with our skin. These free radicals are the very core of the aging process, destroying our body cells one by one.

One of the world's leading nutritionists, Dr. Venket Rao, Professor Emeritus of Nutritional Sciences at the Faculty of Medicine, University of Toronto, has been studying the role of antioxidants and their availability to the body's cells since 1997. When I met him recently he said:

"We have repeatedly shown that the protective antioxidants are only valuable if they are biologically available to the body's cells. Oxidative damage is just like rust on a piece of iron. If you coat the iron with an antioxidant, the surface remains perfect. In the body, antioxidants have the same protective effect on every individual cell. We've studied chemically induced cancers in human colon cells, bone loss, prostate cancer cells, breast cancer cells, and long-term dietary intervention in both bone health and prostate patients, and in all these areas the role of antioxidants like lycopene has been proved extremely effective."

Using Professor Rao's analogy, just think what happens to a wrought-iron garden gate if it isn't painted regularly. The paint flakes off, leaving the iron exposed to the air, and the oxygen attacks, making the gate rust. In time, the rust damages the metal and the gate starts to disintegrate. Exactly the same thing happens in the human body. Free radicals circulate through our bodies constantly, looking for healthy cells to latch on to and attack. They aren't choosy about the cells they injure—lungs or liver, stomach or skin, heart or arteries—they'll have a go at anything.

Our only protection is to stop them dead in their tracks and neutralize their destructive potential. The antioxidant chemicals that we get from food are the body's natural police force, patrolling every nook and cranny on their seek-and-destroy journey. If there aren't enough antioxidants, the free radicals win and you suffer premature aging and disease.

The early research into antioxidants focused on specific components of food: vitamins A, C, and E; protective chemicals that were isolated from red wine, broccoli, and cabbages; and carotenoids from carrots, spinach, and greens. It wasn't long before antioxidant pills made with these ingredients appeared on the market, but pills were only half the story. Even in controlled laboratory experiments, using specific antioxidants did not produce nearly such good results as using fresh fruits and vegetables.

So where do we find the foods richest in these miracle chemicals? You find them at the farmer's market or street market, in your corner store, in the supermarket, or they may even be in your own backyard. They are simple, everyday, inexpensive fruits and vegetables. Of course, all fruits and vegetables are good sources of vitamins such as A, C, and E, but those that are deeply colored—dark green, deep red, purple, yellow, and bright orange—tend to have the highest levels of vitamins and minerals.

The antioxidant properties in the pigments that color these wonderful foods are your best weapon against aging. Researchers have identified around 2,000

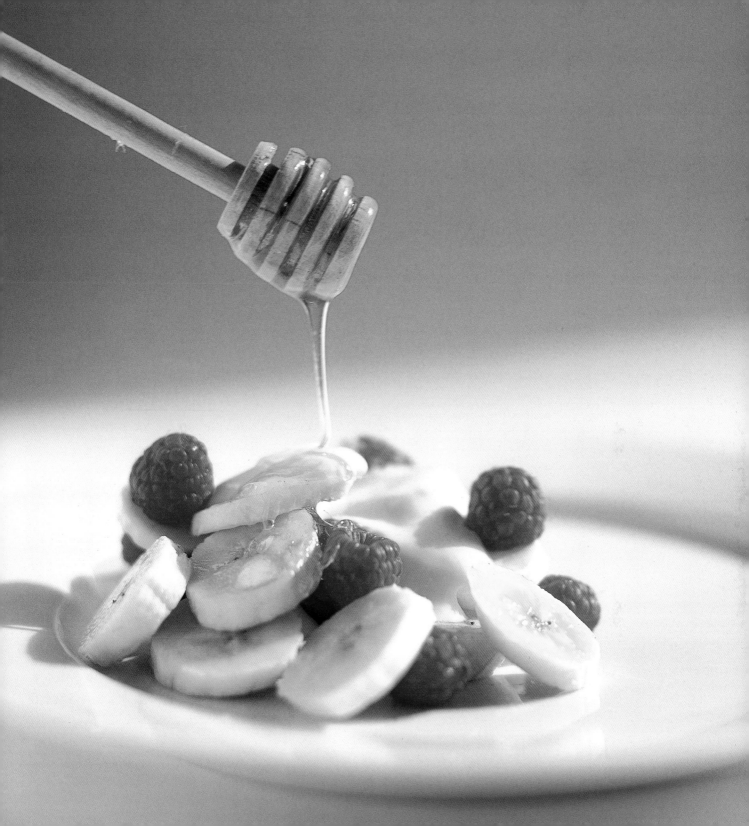

different pigments in plants, including 450 different carotenoids and 150 anthocyanins. These are part of a family of chemicals called polyphenols, which form the most powerfully protective group of natural food chemicals. With such vast numbers of important substances, it's obvious that taking pills, which would contain just a few of the antioxidants, is no match for eating foods that contain them all—though there are specific substances, like beta-carotene for the lungs, lycopene for the heart and prostate, and lutein and xeaxanthine for eye protection, that are valuable supplements.

The ORAC score

The U.S. Department of Agriculture Human Nutrition Research Center on Aging (HNRCA) at Tufts University in Boston has been studying the role of antioxidants for some years now. Because large trials with specific antioxidant vitamins had not been conclusive, scientist Ron Prior and his colleagues decided to examine the antioxidant properties of whole foods. In their natural state, plants contain more than 4,000 potential antioxidant chemicals, and there is strong evidence that these are protective against many life-threatening conditions. Just one study—of 1,300 elderly people in Massachusetts—showed that people who ate two or more portions a day of dark green and yellow vegetables were only half as likely to suffer a fatal heart attack and had a third of the risk of dying of cancer compared with people averaging less than one portion a day.

As always in nature, there is a synergistic benefit from the interaction of all the phytochemicals in the plants we consume, and Prior and his team set out to measure the total antioxidant powers of individual foods. They established the oxygen radical absorbance capacity—the ORAC score—a measure of each food's ability to neutralize free radicals and protect the body from aging, heart disease, cancer, and other degenerative conditions. All plant foods are a source of ORAC, and that includes whole grains, nuts, seeds, and beans as well as fruits and vegetables. Meat, fish, and dairy products have vital nutritional roles, but they do not have a significant ORAC value. The highest scores are found in the most colorful produce, such as blueberries, blackberries, cranberries, kale, strawberries, spinach, Brussels sprouts, beets, and sweet potatoes—not surprisingly, dried fruits, with all the water removed, are weight for weight the richest of all.

The HNRCA has produced a table of high-ORAC foods.

Fruit or vegetable ORAC per 3½ ounces

Fruit or vegetable	ORAC		Fruit or vegetable	ORAC
Prunes	5,770		Corn	400
Raisins	2,830		Eggplant	390
Blueberries	2,400		Cauliflower	377
Blackberries	2,036		Peas, fresh or frozen	364
Garlic	1,939		Potatoes	313
Kale	1,770		Sweet potatoes	301
Cranberries	1,750		Cabbage, raw	298
Strawberries	1,540		Leaf lettuce	262
Spinach	1,260		Cantaloupe	252
Raspberries	1,220		Bananas	221
Brussels sprouts	980		Apples	218
Plums	949		Tofu	213
Alfalfa sprouts	930		Carrots	207
Broccoli	890		Green beans	201
Beets	840		Tomatoes	189
Avocados	782		Zucchini	176
Oranges	750		Apricots	164
Red grapes	739		Peaches	158
Red bell peppers	710		Squash, yellow	150
Cherries	670		Lima beans	136
Kiwi fruit	602		Pears	134
Baked beans	503		Iceberg lettuce	116
Pink grapefruit	483		Watermelon	104
Kidney beans	460		Honeydew melon	97
Onions	450		Celery	61
Green grapes	446		Cucumbers	54

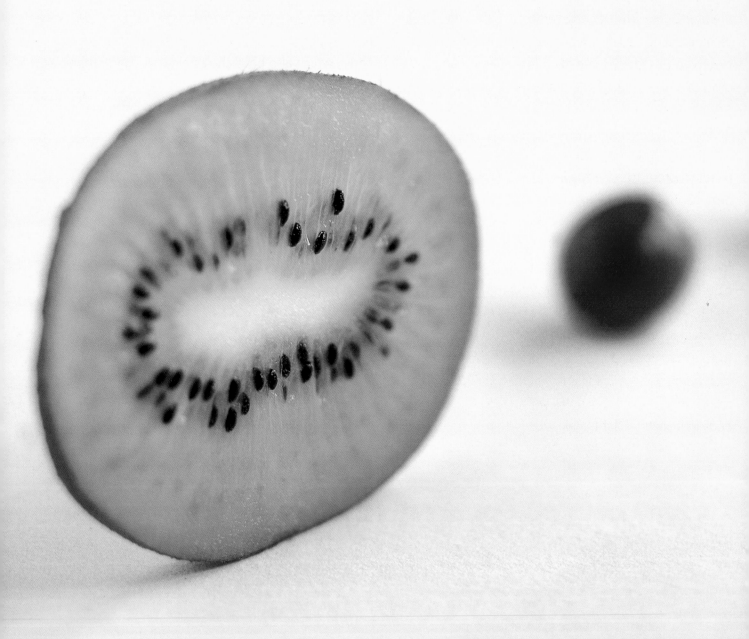

My analysis of hundreds of my patients' diets over the last few years shows that their average daily intake of ORAC units is just over 1,000, and even those on otherwise healthy diets tend to consume far more of the low-ORAC fruits and vegetables. Although these provide adequate supplies of vitamins and minerals, they won't produce the maximum antiaging and protective potential of the high-ORAC foods. According to Prior, we should all be aiming for at least 3,000—and for maximum protection, 5,000—ORAC units every single day. This is the amount your body needs in order to raise the levels of antioxidant protection for every vulnerable cell.

Consistently eating sufficient quantities of high-ORAC foods increases the antioxidant effectiveness of your blood by up to 25 percent. It protects the heart, arteries, and tiniest capillaries of the circulatory system. It slows down aging in the skin. It prolongs effective mental functions and may protect against Alzheimer's disease, multiple sclerosis, and Parkinson's. Most dramatically, following the ORACle diet will, without doubt, help your body in its natural fight against the ravages of cancer.

All of these foods, in addition to their high ORAC value and their key antiaging properties, are also some of the richest sources of other nutrients: folic acid in kale, spinach, Brussels sprouts, and broccoli; vitamin C in blueberries, blackberries, strawberries, raspberries, red bell peppers, oranges, cherries, and kiwi fruit; vitamin E in blackberries, spinach, alfalfa sprouts, and avocados; iron in prunes, raisins, spinach, and beets; bioflavonoids in pink grapefruit, oranges, and cherries; natural antiseptics and antifungals in onions and garlic, which also have cholesterol-lowering properties.

But is it easier to get all the nutrients you need from pills?

Supplements: Do you need them?

At a time when everyone talks about the importance of vitamins and minerals, and they're even listed on your breakfast cereal box, it's hard to believe that it's been less than 100 years since Casimir Funk and Sir Frederick Gowland discovered these essential micronutrients. Now, in the twenty-first century, the shelves in health stores, drugstores, and supermarkets groan under a vast array of supplements.

Multivitamins, single vitamins, megadose mixtures, pills, capsules, and combinations for almost any illness you can think of . . . there are so many variations, it's not surprising that people leave the store confused and empty-handed.

But do you need them anyway?

The answer for a lot of you will be yes—in spite of the fact that most doctors will tell you that you get all you need from your food. In an ideal world, where everyone ate a balanced diet of fresh, homemade meals and used mainly organic ingredients, few of you would benefit from supplements. But the truth is very different.

A recent survey of 800 people in 500 households revealed that the diets of 93 percent of men and 98 percent of women between the ages of eighteen and fifty-four were deficient in folic acid, 60 percent of women were getting too little iron, 90 percent of men and women were getting insufficient amounts of vitamin B6, 73 percent of women were getting less than their minimum requirement of calcium and 50 percent of them weren't getting enough zinc.

I analyze the diets of several hundred patients every year and hardly any of them get enough of all the essential nutrients to meet the minimum daily requirements. They're also commonly short of selenium, iodine, and vitamins E and D. Even the vital vitamin C is often deficient in the diets of men, women, and children.

These nutrient deficiencies can have a devastating effect on health. Many of the world's leading nutritionists believe that although the recommended daily allowances (RDAs) may be enough to prevent deficiency diseases like scurvy, rickets, and beriberi, they're far too low to promote optimum health and protect against disease in general.

Even assuming you get enough nutrients in your food, there are other factors that may keep you from absorbing many of them. For example, spinach is rich in calcium, but because spinach contains chemicals called oxalates, you'll be lucky if 5 percent of it is absorbed. If you take a large dose of iron, zinc, magnesium, or calcium, it can reduce the absorption of the others and mean you need more of them, too.

Eating lots of whole-grain cereals, bran, and soy products can also reduce absorption of minerals. The chemicals in spinach, beets, rhubarb, gooseberries, and chocolate block the absorption of calcium and iron; and strong tea contains tannins, which also interfere with iron absorption. It doesn't help if you drink coffee, as caffeine is a diuretic and makes you lose calcium in your urine. Studies have shown a direct link between coffee drinking and loss of bone density, so it's a good idea to have your morning cereal with milk or your calcium tablet an hour after your first morning coffee.

Phosphorous is another mineral essential for bones, but getting too much of it from cola drinks increases the body's loss of calcium.

Taking huge doses of vitamins isn't the answer either: The more you take, the less your body can absorb. In small doses of vitamin B12, for instance, 70 percent is absorbed, but if you take more than you need, the amount your body actually gets can range from nothing to 50 percent. The same is true for most other B vitamins and vitamin C.

Because zinc is known to help with colds and male fertility, it has become extremely popular as a supplement, but excessive amounts can reduce the quantity of copper in the body and that can lower the levels of the good HDL cholesterol in your blood.

One much ignored and little understood area is the bad effects that many prescribed medicines have on nutritional status. These include appetite suppressants; chemotherapy, which causes nausea or vomiting; laxatives, which reduce all nutrient absorption; aluminum-based antacids, which interfere with the absorption of phosphorus; some epilepsy medications, which can affect folic acid absorption and cause anemia; and cholesterol-lowering drugs, which can reduce the body's levels of vitamins A, D, E, and K.

Antibiotics can also kill the good bacteria responsible for producing B vitamins. Birth-control pills may reduce levels of B6, and diuretics could make you lose potassium, which is essential for all muscles, including the heart. These reactions can be more worrying in people who have a poor diet to start with or serious health problems, and in growing children.

The people who will certainly need to supplement their diets are those who are physically very active, like athletes and dancers—and, worryingly, children and adolescents who live on junk food and refuse all efforts to persuade them to eat fruits and vegetables. Anyone preparing for or recovering from surgery or recuperating from any acute illness, pregnant or breast-feeding women, individuals with stressful personal or business lives, and people with any chronic bowel disorder will also require supplements.

People with mouth or throat problems that prevent normal eating, women past menopause, and, of course, the elderly, whose digestive systems are less efficient and who tend to eat less anyway, are candidates, too. Obviously, supplements are essential in the treatment of eating disorders and for anyone else whose life is so haphazard that regular eating is impossible.

So, of course, vitamin, mineral, and nutritional pills have an important role to play, but far too many people treat them as substitutes for food rather than supplements to a healthy diet. The simple truth is that no one can live on junk food, take a pill, and expect to be healthy.

Food—the secret of youth

There is already a substantial growth in the number of people taking early retirement, and as the population continues to age many of us will have the opportunity to enjoy twenty-five to thirty years of leisure. I suspect that a huge proportion of people will decide to do some part-time work for the mental stimulus as well as the extra money it can provide during these golden years. But to give yourself the fullest sense of well-being and enjoyment in this period of your life, you need to be healthy.

You don't need a revolution in your eating, you don't need rigid or peculiar diets, and you certainly don't need expensive pills and potions—just lots of the foods that look good, taste good, and will do you the ultimate good. These are the foods that will prolong your active years, something that's becoming more important than ever as life expectancy increases and modern medicine extends its ability to keep us alive.

Of course, there are no miracle answers, but if you follow the immensely enjoyable ORACle diet, you give the odds for healthy living an enormous boost in your favor.

Everyone must now know that five portions of fruit and vegetables a day—totaling approximately one pound in weight—is the minimum quantity needed for a well-balanced and healthy diet. But if you really want to beat the aging process and achieve maximum health protection, make it seven portions, at least three of which come from the list of high-ORAC foods. It really is easier than you think. Each of these delicious mixtures will give you optimum high-ORAC protection on a daily basis:

- *1/4 cup prunes, and 1 tablespoon each blueberries and raisins with your breakfast cereal, or*

- *2 1/4 cups spinach, 3/4 cup Brussels sprouts, and a salad with 1/2 red bell pepper, 1 tablespoon alfalfa sprouts, and 1 tablespoon broccoli florets with your midday meal, or*

- *3/4 cup cooked baby beets; a large red bell pepper stuffed with corn, chopped onion, and raisins; and a bowl of cherries or strawberries with dinner*

Boost your levels even more by eating California prunes and raisins as between-meal snacks throughout the day.

The high-ORAC guide is your chance to protect your body from the visible and invisible effects of aging. You can slow down the development of wrinkles and old-looking, pitted skin; protect your joints from arthritis and your nervous system from early dementia and senility; reduce your risks of heart disease; and increase your chances of avoiding many forms of cancer. All you have to do is make sure your nutritional bank balance is always in the red, blue, yellow, orange, and green. This is the food rainbow that will color you healthy.

This must be the simplest and most enjoyable prescription for health and long life that has ever been devised. Each recipe in this book has a star rating, and each star represents 1,000 ORAC units. Take a quick look at the recipes and menus and you'll see how incredibly easy it is to reach and exceed the optimum 5,000. Don't forget that fruit and vegetable juices are excellent ORAC sources, too, and provide almost the same score as whole produce.

You may be surprised that in a healthy-eating book there are no prohibitions or dire warnings about fat, calories, carbohydrates, or sweets. The reason there aren't is not because you can push up your ORACs, stuff yourself with burgers, fries, and candy, and still expect to reap all the benefits. The fact is, by increasing the amount of plant foods in your diet, you will automatically push out a lot of the less healthy foods. It's also important that we all get back to the joy of eating and stop equating pleasure with sin.

Food is not just fuel. It's there to be relished, enjoyed, and, whenever possible, eaten in the good company of friends and family. It's part of the cement that binds social groups together, part of the social structure that helps children learn how to communicate, and, just as important, acquire both knowledge and love of food and cooking.

Where your food is concerned, it's what you do most of the time that matters to your health and well-being. What you do occasionally doesn't matter at all.

Enjoy and be well!
Each recipe in this book has a star rating, with each star representing 1,000 ORAC units.

★	1,000 ORAC units
★★	2,000 ORAC units
★★★	3,000 ORAC units
★★★★	4,000 ORAC units
★★★★★	5,000 ORAC units (optimum)

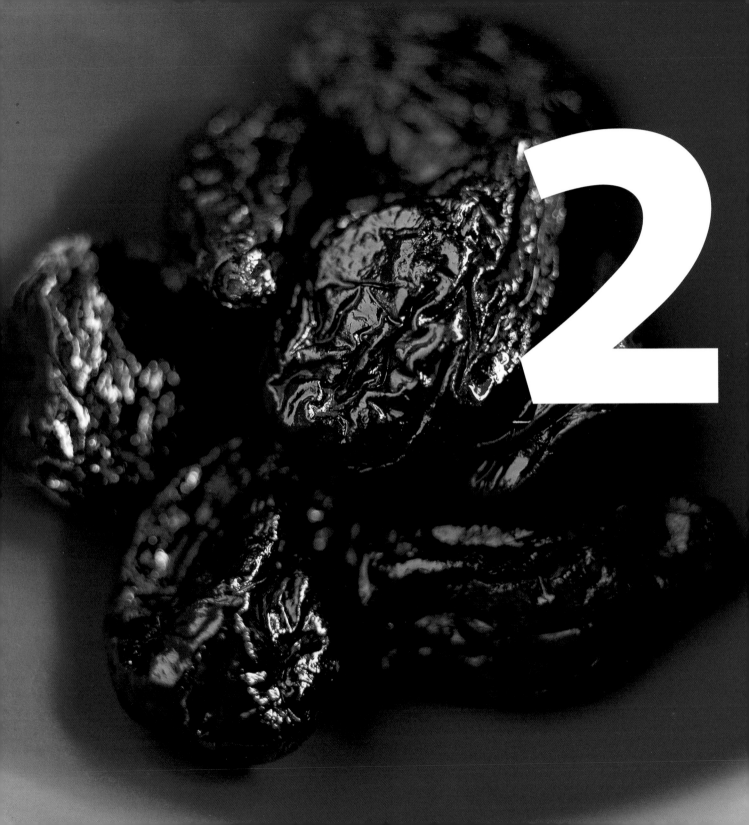

2

breakfasts

All recipes in this chapter serve 2

ORAC value per serving ★★★★★★✔

oatmeal with prunes and apricots

The hardy Scots have known for centuries that oatmeal is the best possible start to the day—and how right they are! Protein, B vitamins, and slow-release energy make this the perfect breakfast. But when you add the dried fruit in this recipe, you get the additional protective benefits of a truly huge ORAC score.

2 cups good organic rolled oats
2 cups milk
2 cups water
8 pitted prunes
8 dried apricots
2 teaspoons organic brown sugar
Extra milk for drizzling

1 Put the rolled oats into a saucepan.

2 Add the milk and water and bring to a gentle simmer, stirring occasionally. Cook for 5 minutes or as directed on the box, adding more milk if the mixture gets too thick.

3 Meanwhile, snip the prunes and apricots to the size of half a teaspoon and add them to the cooked oatmeal. Cover and leave for 1 minute.

4 Pour into two bowls, sprinkle with sugar, and let sit for about 1 minute.

5 Serve with the extra milk drizzled on top.

ORAC value per serving ★★★

fruity appetizer with beans and tomatoes

This is a terrific breakfast that will provide you with four times as much vitamin C as you need for a whole day, 20 percent of your calcium needs, plenty of protein from the beans, whole-wheat bread, and the special type of soluble fiber that all beans contain, which helps lower the cholesterol in your blood. All this before you even think about its super ORAC score.

1 large pink grapefruit
4 kiwi fruit, peeled and sliced
2 tablespoons yogurt sauce (see page 126)
4 fresh tomatoes
2 slices whole-wheat bread
1²/₃ cups canned organic baked beans

1 Peel the grapefruit, leaving some of the pith attached to the fruit, and separate the sections.

2 Arrange the grapefruit and kiwi fruit around the perimeter of two plates and place the yogurt sauce in the middle. Serve while you cook the rest of the meal.

3 Put the tomatoes in one layer in a saucepan of water. Bring to a boil and cook until the skins begin to split—3–5 minutes, depending on size—then strip the skins off.

4 Meanwhile, toast the bread and heat the beans.

5 Serve the tomatoes next to the beans heaped on the toast.

ORAC value per serving ★★✦

"grorange" juice, poached egg, and poached tomato

Masses of vitamin C; lots of lycopene from the tomatoes for prostate- and breast-cancer protection; protein, iron, and B vitamins from the eggs; and fiber from the whole-wheat toast . . . what more could you ask for, apart from a fantastic helping of ORAC?

2 cups freshly squeezed orange juice
1 cup freshly squeezed grapefruit juice
1 teaspoon organic vinegar—the flavor doesn't matter
4 organic free-range eggs
4 tomatoes
2 slices whole-wheat toast

1 Mix the juices in a pitcher and pour into two glasses.

2 Fill a large skillet with water and bring to a simmer. (You may have to cook this breakfast in two batches if your skillet isn't large enough.) Add the vinegar.

3 Roll the eggs, still in their shells, in the water for about 30 seconds (this keeps the whites together as they poach). Remove and set aside for another 30 seconds.

4 Add the tomatoes to the skillet.

5 Break in the eggs and simmer for 4 minutes or until the egg yolks are as firm as you like and the tomato skins start to split.

6 Serve the eggs and tomatoes on slices of whole-wheat toast.

ORAC value per serving ★★✦

avocado with sliced tomato

Avocados are a source of one the healthiest of all oils—monounsaturated fat, which helps reduce cholesterol and blood pressure. They also contain a large amount of vitamin E, which protects the heart and blood vessels and is essential for clean, supple skin. With the vitamin C from the tomatoes and lemon juice, this adds up to a slightly unusual, but extremely healthy, antiaging breakfast with a substantial protective ORAC score.

2 large, ripe, but not bruised, avocados, peeled and pitted
1 tablespoon lemon juice
Freshly ground black pepper
2 slices whole-wheat bread
4 tomatoes, sliced

1 Mash the avocados thoroughly.

2 Add the lemon juice, to prevent the avocados from discoloring, and a few twists of freshly ground black pepper.

3 Toast the bread and heap on the avocado mash.

4 Serve with the sliced tomatoes on the side.

ORAC value per serving ★↙

honeyed fruit and yogurt

Nothing could be quicker than this delicious summer breakfast. Lots of energy and potassium from the bananas; vitamin C from the raspberries; calcium, protein, and immune-boosting good bacteria in the yogurt; and an instant lift from the honey. Perfect if you're going to the gym, for a run, or to play a game of tennis—and a good start to your ORAC day.

2 bananas, peeled and sliced
1 cup raspberries
1 1/4 cups plain live organic yogurt
About 2 tablespoons honey, preferably organic

1 Divide the banana slices between two bowls.

2 Gently wash the raspberries, taking care not to bruise them, and pile on top of the bananas.

3 Tip half the yogurt into each bowl.

4 Drizzle with the honey.

ORAC value per serving ★★★★★

Swiss muesli with blueberries

The traditional alpine start to the day and a far cry from the sawdust texture of cheap muesli with added milk eaten immediately. Good muesli is made with oats and lots of raisins, sultanas, and other dried fruits, so you get instant energy from the fruit sugars, slow-release energy from the oats, calcium and beneficial bacteria from the yogurt, and a huge amount of vitamin C from the blueberries. This is another age-defying breakfast with an abundance of ORACs.

About 3 cups organic apple juice
2 bowls half filled with good-quality, unsweetened, preferably organic muesli
3/4 cup plain live organic yogurt
1 cup fresh blueberries

1 The night before, pour the juice onto the muesli—it should almost drown it, as the cereal mix will nearly double in size—then stir in the yogurt.

2 In the morning, wash the blueberries carefully.

3 Serve the muesli with the blueberries piled on top.

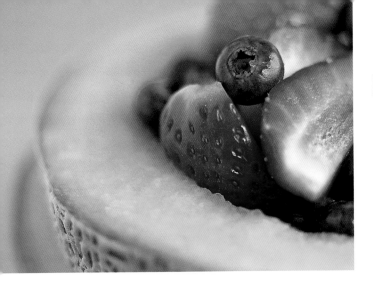

deviled prunes with spicy tomato sauce

Definitely not a Monday-morning breakfast—unless it's a holiday—but a perfect, leisurely weekend brunch. Traditionally, "devils on horseback," made with kidneys, are served as a treat after dinner in the upper-class gentlemen's clubs in London. They became a popular breakfast dish during the days of the British Raj in India. Made here with prunes, they're as delicious as they are dramatically high in their ORAC score.

12 leaves Italian parsley
12 large pitted prunes, washed and
  thoroughly dried
6 large slices organic bacon
1 quantity spicy tomato sauce (see page 123)

1 Place a parsley leaf on top of each prune.

2 Cut most of the fat off the bacon, stretch each slice with the back of a wooden spatula, and cut in half lengthwise. Wrap the bacon around the prunes and parsley and secure with half a toothpick.

3 Put the wrapped prunes on a baking sheet and place under the broiler, turning until the bacon is well cooked but not crispy.

4 Serve with the tomato sauce.

ORAC value per serving ★★★★

fruit-filled melon shells

As breakfast, an appetizer, a dessert, or a lunchtime snack, this is refreshing, tasty, and unbelievably healthy. The melon provides lots of beta-carotene for eyes and skin, and all the berries will give you around five times the amount of vitamin C you need for one day. But the real gift from nature in this recipe is its staggeringly high ORAC score from such a small amount of food.

About 1¹/₄ cups of mixed strawberries, blueberries, blackberries, and red currants
1 ripe cantaloupe, halved and seeded

1 Wash the berries carefully, removing any hulls.

2 Wash the currants and strip them from their stalks, but don't bother to hull them—they are easily digested.

3 Heap the soft fruit into the hollows in the melon and serve.

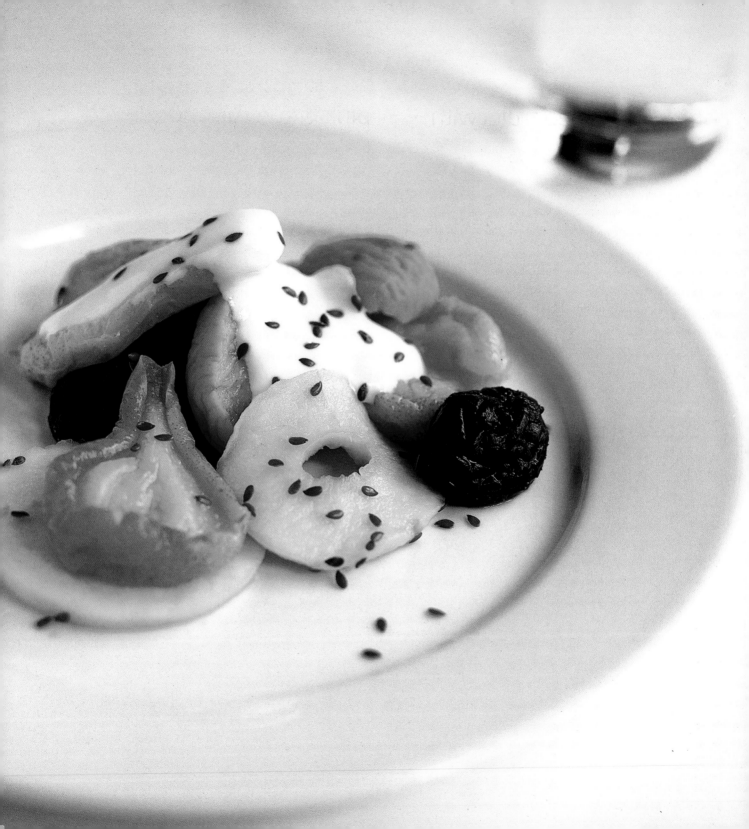

ORAC value per serving ★★★★★★

compote of dried fruits with yogurt and flaxseeds

If you're in a hurry in the morning, this is the healthy alternative to stopping on the way to work for coffee and a doughnut. Prepared the night before, it will take less than five minutes to pour on the yogurt and eat—and it will help get your day off to a flying start. Energy, beta-carotene, fiber, calcium, and masses of vitamin E from the flaxseeds are the extra rewards on top of a huge ORAC score.

2¹/₂ cups mixed dried fruits: pitted prunes, apricots, mangoes, raisins, blueberries, apples, bananas, or any other that you like
1¹/₄ cups plain organic yogurt
2 tablespoons flaxseeds

1 Put the fruit in a large bowl and cover with boiling water. Allow to cool, then refrigerate overnight.

2 In the morning, drain the fruit. Arrange the fruit and yogurt on two plates, sprinkle with the flaxseeds, and serve.

ORAC value per serving

pink grapefruit and stewed herrings with gooseberry sauce

Herrings are a superb source of essential fatty acids and vitamin D. They also provide excellent protein and minerals, including iodine. Despite their salt content, they're a useful heart-protective food as long as you keep your overall salt consumption as low as possible. The gooseberry sauce is an extra luxury that will provide a valuable ORAC addition. Starting with pink grapefruit gives you lots of extra vitamin C and more ORAC.

1 large pink grapefruit
2 naturally smoked, undyed herrings
Gooseberry sauce (see page 124)

1 Halve the grapefruit and cut around the sections.

2 Fill a large pitcher with freshly boiled water. Drop in the herrings, head first. Cover tightly with foil and leave for 7 minutes. Meanwhile, go ahead and enjoy your grapefruit.

3 Pull out the fish by their tails and allow any excess water to drain off. Serve with the sauce.

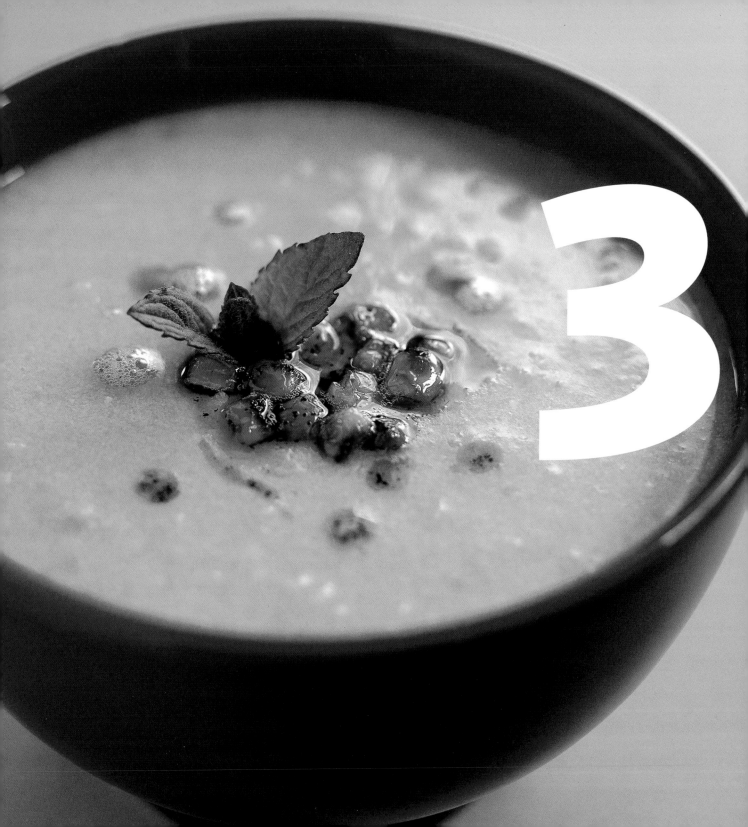

soups

All recipes in this chapter serve 4

ORAC value per serving ★

basic stock

In these days of instant stock cubes and "fresh" stock on the supermarket shelves, the art of making stock is disappearing fast. I think that's a great shame, as none of the commercially prepared stocks tastes as good as your own, and they certainly don't have the ORAC value of this recipe. This stock is easy to make and freezes well—I turn it into ice cubes, which can then be used to enhance stews, casseroles, sauces, and, of course, as the basis for any delicious soup. This is one kitchen skill that handsomely repays such a small investment in time and effort.

2 large onions
2 celery ribs with their leaves, washed
4 leeks, trimmed and washed
4 large carrots, trimmed and peeled
3 tomatoes, quartered
2 sprigs thyme
1 large sprig rosemary
2 bay leaves
6 peppercorns

1 Peel and slice one onion. Leave the other whole and unpeeled—the skin will give extra color to the stock.

2 Put all the ingredients into a large saucepan with about 4¹/₂ quarts of water. A pasta or asparagus pan with a steamer or strainer inside is ideal.

3 Simmer gently, uncovered, for 2 hours. Remove the vegetables from the pan and push through a strainer into the stock.

ORAC value per serving ★ ✈

sweet potato and pear

This is a robust soup, which doesn't need liquidizing, although I like to mash the pears and sweet potatoes gently with a fork before serving. As well as its benefits for anyone with urinary tract infections (thanks to the cranberry juice) and its very high content of cancer-protective beta-carotenes, it also has an unusual flavor and a high ORAC score.

2 tablespoons extra-virgin olive oil
1 large red onion or 2 smaller ones, chopped
4 sweet potatoes, peeled and cubed
5 conference pears, peeled, cored, and cubed
1 cup cranberry juice
3³/₄ cups basic stock (see previous recipe)
¹/₂ teaspoon ground nutmeg, preferably fresh
1¹/₄ cups plain organic yogurt

1 Heat the oil in a large saucepan, add the onions, and sauté gently for 5 minutes.

2 Add the sweet potatoes and pears to the pan with the cranberry juice and stock.

3 Bring to a boil and simmer for 45 minutes.

4 Crush the vegetables roughly with a potato masher.

5 Stir in the nutmeg and yogurt.

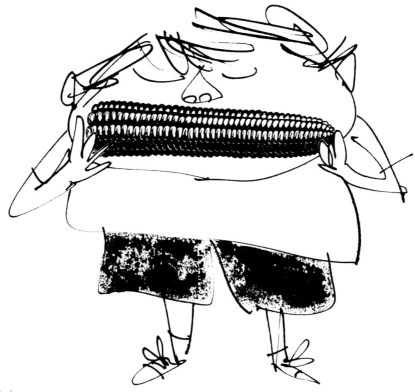

ORAC value per serving ★ ◢

minty pea and corn

This wonderful summer soup takes a little longer to prepare than opening and heating a can of soup, or, even worse, using one of the instant soup powders full of salt and chemicals. It's an interesting variation on ordinary pea soup, providing extra calcium from the cream cheese, a delicious creamy texture, and a good ORAC score.

1 cup frozen peas
1 cup frozen corn
3 cups basic stock (see page 30)
6 large sprigs mint
11/4 cups low-fat cream cheese, softened
3 large sprigs fresh chervil or 1/2 teaspoon dried
Salt and pepper
1/4 cup unsalted butter

1 Cook the peas and 3/4 cup of the corn in the stock with two sprigs of mint until tender—about 5 minutes.

2 Stir in the cream cheese, chervil, and two more mint sprigs and heat gently for 2 minutes.

3 Puree in batches in a blender until very smooth. Leave to cool, then put in the refrigerator to chill.

4 Check seasoning, adding freshly ground pepper or salt if necessary.

5 Sauté the remaining corn in the butter, then sprinkle on the soup.

6 Serve with remaining mint and chervil leaves (if you have them) floating on top.

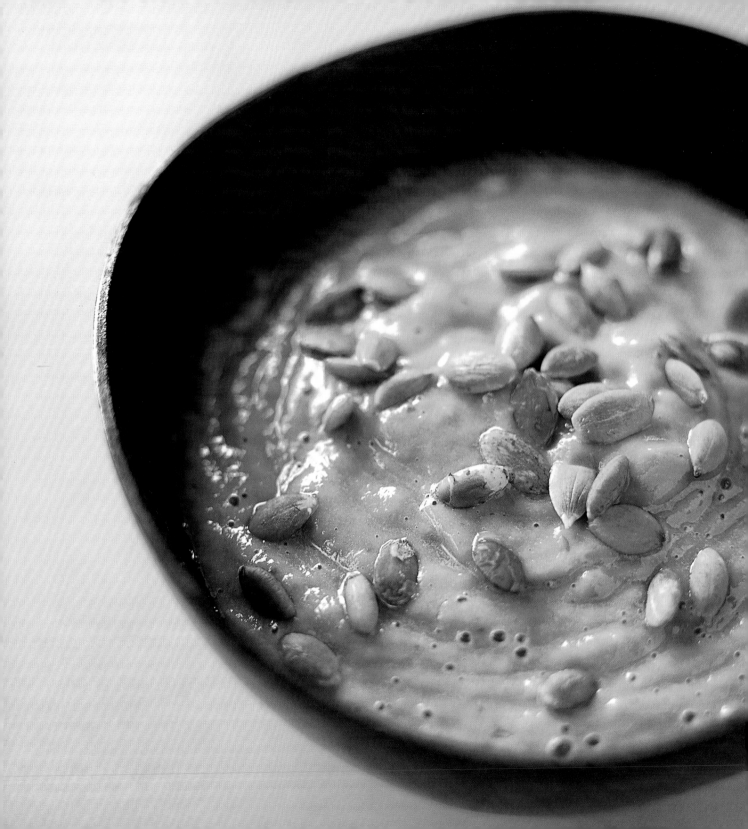

ORAC value per serving ★★★

chilled avocado

A bowl of this will do more for your skin than a fortune's worth of fancy cosmetics. Antiaging, wrinkle-beating, and highly protective against heart disease, circulation problems, and cancer, the smooth, cool appearance belies the hot spiciness of these Mexican flavors. A single bowl contains more than half your daily ORAC requirement.

5 ripe avocados, peeled and pitted
4^1/$_2$ cups chicken stock from the real chicken soup recipe (see page 40)
3 tablespoons lemon juice
2 large garlic cloves, finely chopped
3 red chilies, seeded and chopped
^{1}/$_4$ teaspoon cayenne pepper
4 plump scallions, roughly chopped
Leaves of 12 large stems cilantro
1 cup canned organic plum tomatoes, drained
^{2}/$_3$ cup plain organic yogurt
^{1}/$_4$ cup pumpkin seeds
Salt and pepper

1 Put the avocado into a food processor with the chicken stock and add the lemon juice.

2 Add the garlic, chilies, and cayenne pepper and blend until smooth.

3 Add the scallions, cilantro leaves, and tomatoes and process briefly again.

4 Add the yogurt and process for just a few seconds. Season to taste and leave in the refrigerator to chill.

5 Dry-fry the pumpkin seeds gently and allow to cool. Serve the soup with the pumpkin seeds floating on top.

ORAC value per serving ★★

carrot and coconut

This combination of mundane carrots and exotic coconut with the spiciness of cilantro is reminiscent of tropical islands. For many people, just the smell of coconut makes them think of sunshine and blue seas. This soup will certainly put the sunshine back into your life.

2 tablespoons extra-virgin olive oil
1 large onion, finely chopped
2 pounds carrots, diced
^{1}/$_2$ teaspoon coriander
3 cups basic stock (see page 30)
1^3/$_4$ cups canned coconut milk
Salt and pepper
2 sprigs cilantro

1 Heat the oil in a large saucepan, add the onion, and sauté for 5 minutes.

2 Add the carrots to the pan with the coriander and continue cooking for 10 minutes, stirring constantly.

3 Pour in the stock and coconut milk and simmer until the carrots are tender—this shouldn't take more than 10 minutes.

4 Puree in a food processor until smooth, then reheat and season to taste.

5 Tear the leaves from the cilantro sprigs and serve the soup with the leaves floating on top.

ORAC value per serving ★★❯

cheat's gazpacho

Here's another summer favorite, which brings back memories of vacations in Spain. The best I've ever had was in a beachside café at the southern resort of Nerja, and I only have to taste gazpacho to smell the wood fire under the chef's paella pan. This quick and easy version is equally delicious and overflows with age-defying ORAC properties.

1 red bell pepper, halved and seeded
1 yellow bell pepper, halved and seeded
1 large sweet Spanish onion, finely chopped
3 garlic cloves, finely chopped
1 large tomato, roughly chopped
1 cucumber, peeled, halved, and seeded
Leaves of 5 large stems cilantro, chopped
4¹/₂ cups good-quality tomato juice
1 tablespoon hot pepper sauce
Salt and pepper
Extra vegetables and cilantro leaves for garnish (optional)

1 Preheat the oven to 350°F. Place the peppers cut side down on a baking sheet and bake in the oven 20 minutes or until the skins begin to wrinkle. When they are cool enough to handle, rub off the skins.

2 Put the other vegetables and the chopped cilantro leaves into a food processor with ¹/₂ cup of the tomato juice. Process briefly so that the consistency is still quite rough.

3 Add the remaining juice and blend at a low speed for 30 seconds. Pour into a pitcher and leave in the refrigerator until cold.

4 When ready to serve, add the hot pepper sauce, then season to taste.

5 Serve garnished with chopped tomato, peeled cucumber cubes, diced peppers, diced onion, and cilantro leaves.

ORAC value per serving ★

greens galore

This is one of my favorite soups, and I've made it here with baby spinach. The idea comes from the wonderful cooking writer Patricia Wells, whose recipe for sorrel soup came from a German chef (sorrel is widely grown in Germany). I grow sorrel in my garden—it thrives like a weed—but it's quite difficult to find in most supermarkets. What a shame! However, the soup can also be made with watercress, chard, dandelion leaves, young stinging nettles, or a combination of all these healthy green leaves.

3 cups baby spinach
¹/₄ cup slightly softened unsalted butter
2 tablespoons extra-virgin olive oil
2 plump scallions, sliced
1 cup peeled and diced potatoes
4¹/₂ cups basic stock (see page 30)
1 cup heavy cream
Salt and pepper
12 chives, snipped

1 Put the washed spinach and butter into a food processor and puree until smooth. Set aside in a cool place.

2 Heat the oil gently in a large saucepan, add the scallions, and sauté gently for 5 minutes.

3 Add the potatoes and cook gently, stirring occasionally, until the potatoes are colored—about 10 minutes. Add the stock and simmer until the potatoes are tender.

4 Stir in the cream. Puree with a hand blender or process in batches in the rinsed-out food processor.

5 If using a food processor, put the mixture back into the saucepan. Season to taste.

6 Whisk the spinach puree into the hot soup and sprinkle with the chives.

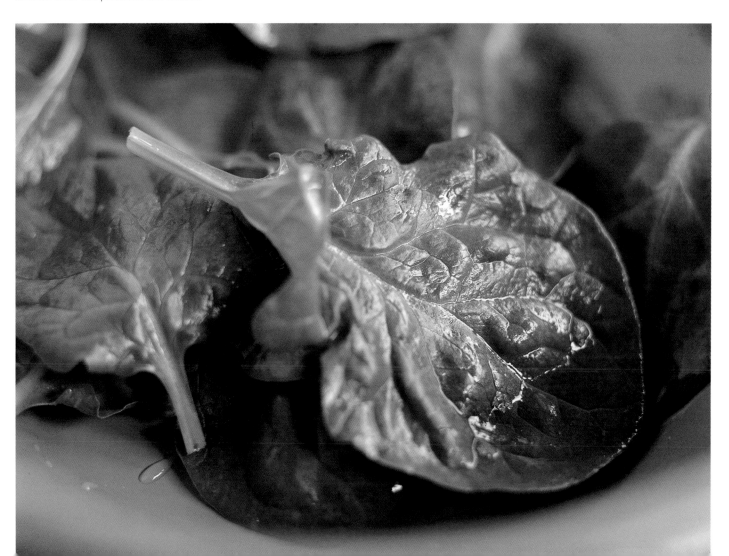

mussel chowder

This recipe may look long, but it's very easy. I don't like mussels, but I love cooking this dish for friends; watching them enjoy it is reward enough for the small amount of effort involved. The chowder is full of essential fatty acids, rich in iodine, and you don't need to worry about the heavy cream—it's only ¼ cup per person, and enjoying good food is essential to good health. Add some good bread and a tomato and onion salad, and you've got a complete meal and an extra dose of ORAC.

3 pounds 5 ounces fresh mussels
6¼ cups mixed dry white wine and basic stock
  (see page 30)
1⅓ cups peeled and finely cubed potatoes
½ cup unsalted butter
2 onions, finely chopped
2 garlic cloves, finely chopped
2 tablespoons all-purpose flour
4 bay leaves
2 large sprigs thyme
5¼ cups baby spinach
½ cup thawed frozen corn
12 large stems Italian parsley
1 cup heavy cream

1 Wash the mussels, discarding any that are open, and pull off the beards. Put them in a large saucepan with the wine and stock.

2 Simmer for 10 minutes. Drain through a large strainer lined with cheesecloth, reserving the cooking liquid. Discard any shells that aren't open and shuck the rest.

3 Boil the potatoes in a separate saucepan for 10 minutes. Drain.

4 Meanwhile, melt the butter in a large saucepan. Add the onions and garlic and sauté gently for 5 minutes.

5 Stir in the flour and continue cooking, stirring continuously, for 2 minutes.

6 Pour in the wine and stock mixture, add the bay leaves and thyme, and simmer for 10 minutes.

7 Tear the spinach roughly and add to the pan with the corn, drained potatoes, and mussels.

8 Reserve eight parsley leaves and finely chop the rest. Add the chopped parsley to the pan and simmer gently for 5 minutes.

9 Stir in the cream and heat through. Serve the chowder with the reserved parsley on top.

ORAC value per serving ★★★

tomato, pepper, and pasta

This is another great one-pot meal—filling, full of vitamins and minerals, and an excellent source of ORAC units. If you can find them, the long, pointed, slightly misshapen peppers always seem to have more flavor.

1/4 cup extra-virgin olive oil
1 red bell pepper, seeded and cut into chunks
1 green bell pepper, seeded and cut into chunks
1 yellow bell pepper, seeded and cut into chunks
1 red onion, finely sliced
3 garlic cloves, finely chopped
1 tablespoon tomato paste
3 3/4 cups basic stock (see page 30)
4 large sprigs thyme
2 large sprigs fresh rosemary
2 cups canned chopped organic plum tomatoes
10 ounces pasta gnocchi or the potato-based variety
   if you prefer
1/4 cup freshly grated Parmesan cheese

1 Heat the oil in a large saucepan, add the peppers, onion, and garlic, and sauté for 10 minutes, stirring regularly.

2 Mix in the tomato paste thoroughly.

3 Pour in the stock, add the thyme and rosemary as whole sprigs, and bring to a boil.

4 Add the chopped tomatoes and simmer for 5 minutes.

5 Remove the sprigs of herbs, put the soup into a food processor in batches, puree until smooth, and return to a clean saucepan.

6 Bring back to a simmer, add the gnocchi, and heat for as long as instructed on the package.

7 Serve the soup sprinkled with the Parmesan cheese.

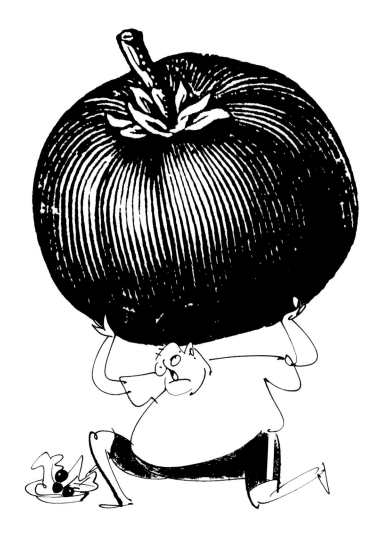

ORAC value per serving ★ ╯

one-pot fish

This mixture of vegetables and fish produces a hearty, stewlike soup that is rich in protein, vitamins, and minerals and contains very little fat. It's a perfect meal for anyone with heart problems or arthritis.

To make your own fish stock, simmer fish trimmings with onion, fresh herbs, and garlic. Some supermarket fish counters will set the trimmings aside for you if you call a day in advance; many independent fish stores do it as a matter of course.

1 parsnip, cubed
8 small new potatoes
1/4 cup unsalted butter
1 sweet onion, very finely chopped
2 garlic cloves, very finely chopped
1 large or 2 small leeks, finely sliced
2 celery ribs, finely sliced
3 tablespoons all-purpose flour
9 cups homemade fish stock (see above) or basic stock
   (see page 30)
About 1 pound 2 ounces mixed cod, turbot, salmon, haddock,
   or your favorite fish, cut into bite-size chunks
8 large sprigs dill, chopped
Freshly ground black pepper
1/2 green cabbage, such as Savoy, very finely chopped
1 cup frozen peas
3 pinches dried saffron

1 Put the parsnip and potatoes into a saucepan of water and boil for 15 minutes until nearly tender.

2 Meanwhile, heat the butter in a saucepan and sauté the onion and garlic for 3 minutes.

3 Add the leeks and celery and continue cooking gently for an additional 3 minutes.

4 Stir in the flour, mix thoroughly, and cook for 2 minutes.

5 Add the stock gradually, stirring continuously to ensure it remains smooth, and keep at simmering point.

6 Drain the parsnip and potatoes and add to the stock.

7 Season the fish with the dill and black pepper and set aside.

8 Add the cabbage to the pan with the peas and saffron and continue to simmer for 5 minutes.

9 Add the fish and continue simmering for an additional 5 minutes, until the fish is just tender.

ORAC value per serving ★★★★

chilled cherry

A favorite from eastern Europe, where luscious cherries grow in abundance. They're not only an extremely rich source of vitamin C, but also contain a group of naturally occurring chemicals called bioflavonoids, which protect the inner walls of your veins and arteries. The combination of cherries and prune juice gives this recipe an extremely high ORAC score, and the sweetness of the wine adds to the complexity of its taste.

3¹/₂ cups fresh pitted cherries
1 cup prune juice
1 cup sweet white wine, such as Sauternes
3 tablespoons honey
2 tablespoons arrowroot

1 Put all but four of the cherries into a processor and puree until smooth. Press firmly through a strainer to remove any skin and to extract the juices.

2 Put the prune juice, white wine, and honey into a saucepan. Heat gently until the honey is fully dissolved.

3 Add the cherry puree and heat gently.

4 Meanwhile, put the arrowroot into a small bowl and mix in just enough water to make a thick, smooth paste. Mix it into the soup and continue heating very gently until the soup starts to thicken. Remove from the heat, leave to cool, then chill in the refrigerator.

5 Halve the remaining four cherries, float them on the soup, and serve.

ORAC value per serving ★★★

easy tomato

Homemade tomato soup in less than 30 minutes—what could be easier? It not only tastes good, but the essential oils in the basil are powerful mood enhancers, so it makes you feel good, too. Not surprisingly, this recipe also does you good, as it is super-rich in beta-carotenes and cancer-preventive lycopene, and has a high ORAC score as well.

3 tablespoons olive oil
1 onion, finely sliced
3 garlic cloves, chopped
2 celery ribs, finely sliced
2 tablespoons sun-dried tomato paste
3 cups basic stock (see page 30)
2 medium roasted bell peppers, drained and sliced if necessary
1 large sprig rosemary
3¹/₂ cups canned organic whole plum tomatoes
Salt and pepper
12 basil leaves

1 Heat the oil in a saucepan, add the onion and garlic, and sauté gently until soft—about 5 minutes.

2 Add the celery and cook for an additional 5 minutes.

3 Stir in the sun-dried tomato paste and combine thoroughly.

4 Add the stock, peppers, rosemary, and tomatoes with their juices and simmer gently for 15 minutes.

5 Remove the rosemary, adjust the seasoning, and serve sprinkled with the whole basil leaves.

ORAC value per serving ★↗

real chicken

Thanks to the special amino acids in chicken soup, this really does have a penicillin-like effect. Of course it's delicious at any time, but for people who are sick or convalescing, it also provides immune-boosting properties. It's not particularly high in ORAC value, but when combined with the other benefits, this is a double-whammy recipe.

1 leftover cooked chicken carcass
1 large onion, unpeeled and quartered
3 bay leaves
6 whole peppercorns
1 bouquet garni
2 large carrots, diced
1/2 rutabaga, diced
1 parsnip, diced
2 small turnips, diced
1 sweet potato, peeled and diced
Salt and freshly ground black pepper

1 Put the chicken carcass into a large saucepan and cover with about 5 1/4 cups of water.

2 Add the onion, bay leaves, peppercorns, and bouquet garni to the pan, bring to a boil, and simmer, covered, for 2 hours. Strain and return the broth to the pan.

3 Add the carrot, rutabaga, parsnip, turnip, and sweet potato to the broth, bring back to a boil, and simmer until the vegetables are tender—about 30 minutes.

4 Season to taste.

ORAC value per serving ★★

cream of broccoli and Brussels sprouts

This is one sure way to get youngsters to eat Brussels sprouts and broccoli, although it's probably best to omit the almonds for young children, just in case of allergies. This is an immensely cancer-protective soup, as these vegetables are exceptionally rich in anticancer plant chemicals. Not surprisingly, the ORAC score is quite high.

3 tablespoons extra-virgin olive oil
1 onion, finely chopped
5 1/4 cups basic stock (see page 30)
2 broccoli heads, cut into florets
3 cups Brussels sprouts, halved
1 bouquet garni
1 heaping cup ground almonds
1 1/4 cups light cream
1/4 cup slivered almonds

1 Heat the oil in a large saucepan. Add the onion and sauté for 5 minutes. Add the stock and bring to a boil.

2 Add the broccoli, Brussels sprouts, bouquet garni, and ground almonds. Simmer gently until the vegetables are just tender, 10–15 minutes.

3 Remove the bouquet garni and liquidize the soup, in batches, in a food processor. Return to the pan.

4 Stir in the cream and heat through. Serve sprinkled with the slivered almonds.

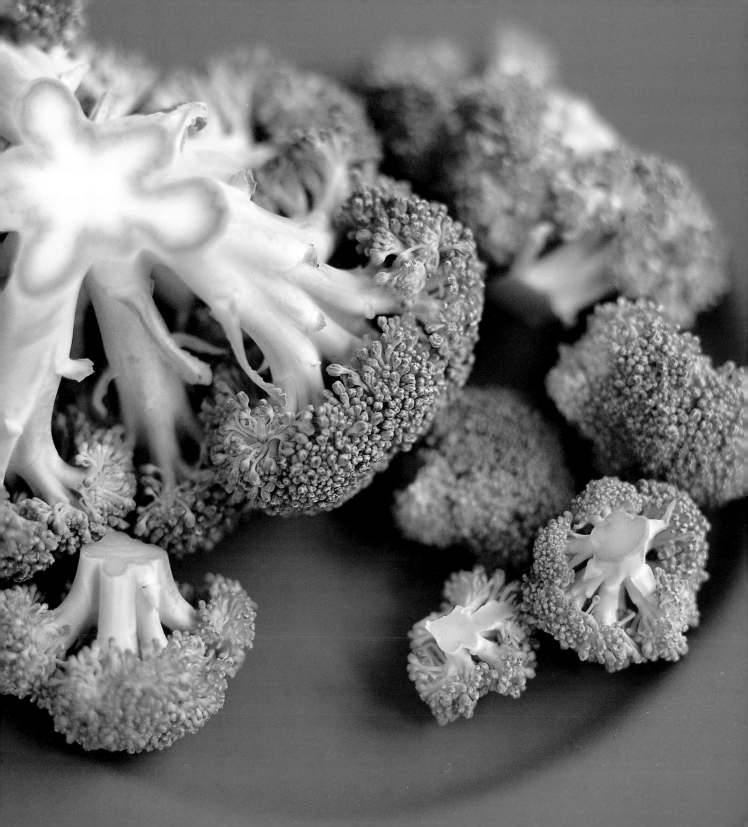

ORAC value per serving ★↗

black bean

My first taste of this soup was on a hot, humid night in the middle of the rainy season chugging up the Amazon in a small boat. The Brazilian woman doing the cooking was a magician with beans—a staple food in that part of South America. She used far more chilies and garlic than I do in this recipe, but surprisingly the intense sweating that her thick dish of soup produced was quite cooling in the tropical heat. The recipe works just as well with haricot, flageolet, or cranberry beans, but it doesn't look quite as dramatic.

3/4 cup dried black beans
6 1/4 cups basic stock (see page 30) or chicken stock from the
   chicken soup recipe (see page 40)
12 stems savory
4 bay leaves
1/4 cup canola oil
1 large onion, finely sliced
4 garlic cloves, finely sliced
3 red chilies, seeded and chopped
1 3/4 cups canned organic tomatoes, coarsely chopped

1 Rinse the beans thoroughly. If using black beans, put into a saucepan of cold water, bring to a boil, and boil for 10 minutes. Drain.

2 Rinse the saucepan, return the beans, and add the stock, savory, and bay leaves. Cover and simmer until tender—this could take a couple of hours. Add extra stock or water if too much of the liquid evaporates.

3 Heat the oil in a deep skillet and sauté the onion, garlic, and chilies for 5 minutes.

4 Add the tomatoes and continue cooking, stirring well, until combined.

5 Stir the contents of the skillet into the beans and stock. Simmer for 5 minutes, then strain, reserving the stock. Remove the bay leaves.

6 Liquidize the beans and vegetables, in batches if necessary, with a ladleful of stock.

7 Return all the pureed vegetables and stock to a clean pan, stir, and heat through.

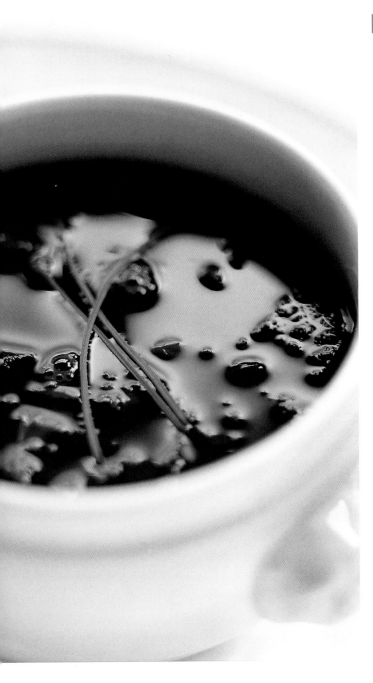

ORAC value per serving

cabbage and beet

Throughout Europe, cabbage is known as the medicine of the poor—and with good reason. It's rich in vitamin C and antibacterial sulfur as well as containing large amounts of cancer-protective plant chemicals. The beet, a seriously undervalued vegetable, is excellent for blood conditions like anemia, and in eastern Europe is traditionally given to people with leukemia. This peasant soup from Poland looks beautiful, tastes delicious, and will do you more good than a bottle of vitamin pills.

1/4 cup canola oil
1 onion, finely chopped
1 garlic clove, finely chopped
1 pound raw baby beets, diced
41/2 cups basic stock (see page 30)
2 tablespoons cider vinegar
3 cups coarsely shredded white cabbage
8 chives

1 Heat the oil in a large saucepan, add the onion and garlic, and sauté for 5 minutes.

2 Mix in the beets, pour in the stock, and boil until tender. Puree in a blender with the cider vinegar and return to the saucepan.

3 Sprinkle the cabbage on the soup, but don't stir. Cover and boil gently for 5 minutes, until the cabbage is almost cooked but still crunchy.

4 Serve with chives arranged on top.

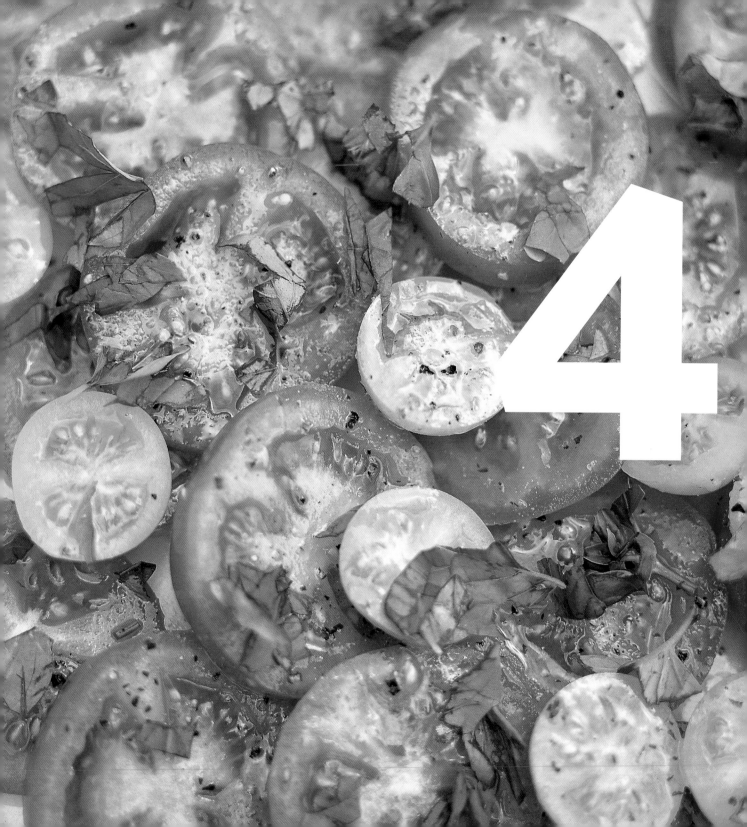

salads

All recipes in this chapter serve 4 unless otherwise stated

ORAC value per serving ★★

beet, pink grapefruit, and red onion

The visual appeal of these wonderful colors is enough to make you feel good before you even taste this dish. But when you add the blood benefits of beets, the heart-protective qualities from the grapefruit, and the disease-fighting chemicals in onions, you really have good health on a plate.

4 small, cooked beets, sliced
2 pink grapefruits, peeled and divided into segments
2 red onions, sliced
1 quantity creamy yogurt dressing (see page 133)

1 Arrange the salad ingredients alternately around the sides of four plates or in a salad bowl.

2 Pour the dressing on top and serve.

ORAC value per serving ★

roasted beets on a bed of red lettuce

This recipe brings out all the flavors of beets, enhanced with the antibacterial, antiviral, and antifungal properties of garlic, and the spicy taste of mustard and good olive oil.

5 tablespoons unsalted butter
8 baby beets, trimmed and rinsed, keeping skins intact
1/4 cup extra-virgin olive oil
2 large scallions, finely chopped
2 tablespoons lime juice
2 garlic cloves, finely chopped
1/2 teaspoon dry mustard
1 large head radicchio or other red lettuce

1 Preheat the oven to 400°F.

2 Cut eight pieces of foil large enough to envelop the beets and rub each piece with butter. Wrap a piece of foil around each beet. Place the beets in the oven and bake for about 1 hour and 15 minutes.

3 Meanwhile, make the dressing. Put the olive oil in a mixing bowl. Add the scallions, lime juice, garlic, and mustard and whisk well. Set aside to let the flavors intermingle.

4 When the beets are cool enough to handle, but still warm, remove from the foil, rub off the skins, and slice.

5 Arrange the lettuce leaves on four plates, lay the beet slices on top, drizzle with the dressing, and serve.

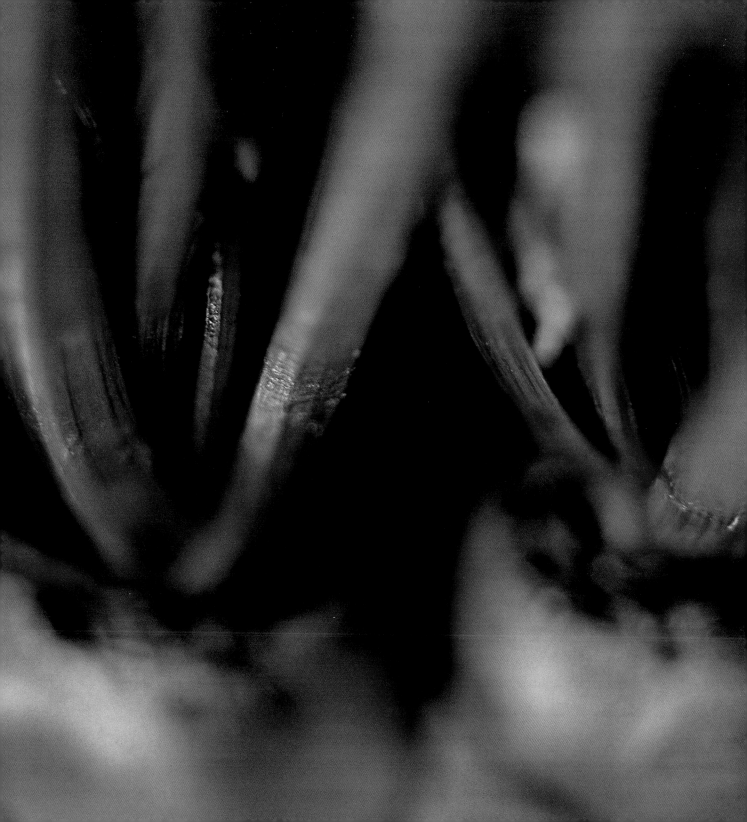

ORAC value per serving ★★

Middle Eastern couscous salad

Cooking the couscous in homemade stock immediately adds to the ORAC score of this salad. Including the cleansing properties of asparagus and the huge beta-carotene content of sun-dried tomatoes with the medicinal benefits of the fresh herbs results in a highly nutritious salad with an excellent ORAC score.

3/4 cup couscous
2 cups basic stock (see page 30) or stock from the
    chicken soup (see page 40)
2 1/4 cups chopped sun-dried tomatoes
1/4 cup extra-virgin olive oil
1 zucchini, diced
1 red bell pepper, seeded and diced
12 fresh asparagus tips
1/4 cup mixed soft herbs, such as Italian parsley, tarragon,
    chervil, and oregano, finely chopped
2 large tomatoes, sliced

1 Put the couscous into a large saucepan with the stock and cook according to package instructions.

2 Meanwhile, soak the sun-dried tomatoes in freshly boiled water for 2 minutes and snip into 1/2 inch strips.

3 Heat the oil in a skillet and gently sauté the zucchini, pepper, asparagus, and tomatoes for 5 minutes.

4 Put the couscous into a bowl and mix in the sautéed vegetables.

5 Stir the herbs into the couscous and top with the sliced tomatoes.

ORAC value per serving ★★

wild and red rice on radicchio

The wonderful red color in the Camargue rice contrasts beautifully with the blackness of wild rice. And serving each portion inside a whole head of radicchio is certainly eye-catching. The dried apricots, cherries, and raisins provide instant energy from their fruit sugars, as well as essential minerals and plenty of fiber.

1/2 cup Camargue rice
3/4 cup wild rice
4 small heads radicchio, trimmed and thoroughly washed
1/3 cup dried cherries, snipped
1/2 cup dried apricots, snipped
1/3 cup raisins
1/2 cup chopped walnuts
1 quantity standard French dressing (see page 132)

1 Cook the two rices in separate saucepans, following the package instructions. Drain if necessary and leave to cool.

2 Meanwhile, open the crowns of the radicchio carefully.

3 Mix the cherries and apricots with the raisins and walnuts.

4 Mix the rices together. Add the fruits and nuts and stir until combined.

5 Pour on the dressing and stir thoroughly.

6 Put the rice, fruit, and nut mixture into the center of the radicchio.

ORAC value per serving ★

traditional salade niçoise

This is the ubiquitous recipe from the south of France, and is ideal reminiscence therapy. If you've ever eaten it under the Mediterranean sun, you need only one sniff of its distinctive aroma to transport you back to the sidewalk café and happy memories. Lots of essential fatty acids and bone-building vitamin D from the fish, and carbohydrate, protein, vitamins A and C, iron, and other minerals from the rest of the ingredients make this a complete meal.

1/2 pound new potatoes
4 organic free-range eggs
1 cup green beans, trimmed
1 large head romaine lettuce
3/4 cup drained canned tuna
1/2 cucumber, peeled, seeded, and cut into julienne strips
4 plum tomatoes, coarsely chopped
1/2 cup drained canned anchovy fillets
10 pitted black olives, halved
1/2 quantity standard French dressing (see page 132)

1 Scrub the potatoes and boil until tender. Halve and leave to cool.

2 Semi hard-boil the eggs, simmering for 6 minutes and rinse under cold running water to prevent discoloring. Peel and quarter when they're cool enough to handle.

3 Simmer the beans until just tender, let cool, then cut into 1 inch sticks.

4 Separate the lettuce leaves and place in a large bowl. Pile on the potatoes and beans.

5 Flake the tuna and arrange over the beans. Add the cucumber, tomatoes, and quartered eggs. Arrange the anchovies on top of the eggs.

6 Sprinkle with the olives and pour the dressing on top.

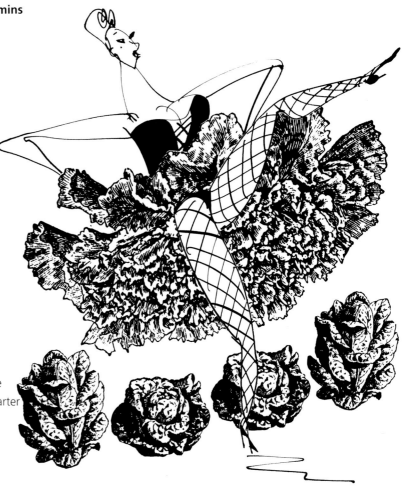

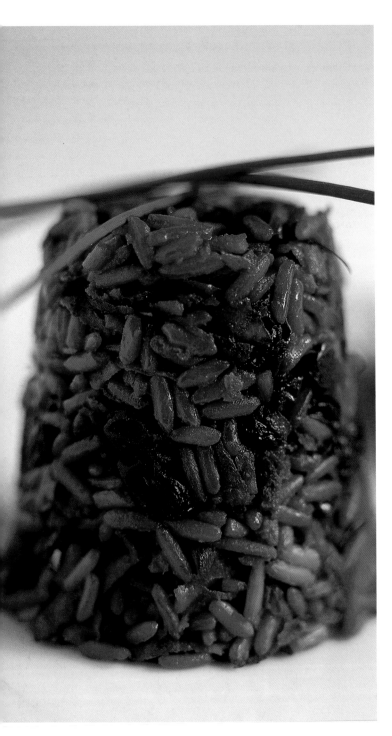

ORACle timbale

A substantial salad that combines the crunchy sweetness of carrots, the heat of the radish, and the unmistakable flavor of celery root. Extra iron from the raisins and the blood-building red pigments in beets make this good to eat at any time, but they're especially useful if you're recovering from an illness or operation.

1 large carrot, trimmed, peeled, and shredded
1 mouli (white radish), trimmed, peeled, and shredded
1/2 celery root, trimmed, peeled, and shredded
2 beets, trimmed, peeled, and shredded
3 cups cooked basmati rice
2 tablespoons finely chopped Italian parsley
1 tablespoon finely snipped chives
2/3 cup raisins
2 tablespoons extra-virgin olive oil
8 whole chives

1 Mix the shredded vegetables thoroughly with the cooked rice.

2 Add the parsley, snipped chives, raisins, and olive oil and stir again.

3 Firmly press the mixture into four timbale pots and refrigerate for at least 1 hour before turning out.

4 Garnish with the whole chives.

ORAC value per serving ★★✔

warm chicken livers with berries

Now that nobody gets their chicken liver inside the bird, you can buy them packaged in virtually any supermarket. You may have to look further for organic livers, but it's worth the effort. As well as massive amounts of vitamins A and B12, you'll get plenty of iron, lots of vitamin C, and a high ORAC score.

3 cups organic chicken livers
2 tablespoons olive oil
2 tablespoons unsalted butter
1 large sprig rosemary
2 garlic cloves, finely chopped
1/2 head romaine lettuce
1/2 head red frisée lettuce
3 large scallions, finely chopped
12 cherry tomatoes, halved
1 cup mixed blackberries and blueberries
1/2 quantity standard French dressing (see page 132)

1 Wash the chicken livers and snip off any pieces of fat or membrane.

2 Heat the oil and butter in a skillet and sauté the livers with the rosemary and garlic, until cooked but still soft—this should take about 5 minutes. Remove the rosemary.

3 Meanwhile, separate the romaine and frisée lettuce leaves and put into a large salad bowl. Mix in the scallions.

4 Put the tomatoes around the sides of the lettuce. Spoon the chicken livers into the middle, reserving the cooking juices, and sprinkle with the blueberries and blackberries.

5 Put the salad dressing into a cold pitcher. Add the reserved cooking juices and mix well. Pour over the salad and serve.

ORAC value per serving ★✔

tabbouleh with a difference

The mixture of bulgur wheat, cucumber, and mint is what gives this dish its distinctly Middle Eastern flavor. But it's the blueberries that account for its high ORAC score. This salad also provides large amounts of vitamin C well in excess of your daily requirement.

3/4 cup bulgur wheat
1 cucumber, peeled, seeded, and diced
1 large red onion, very finely chopped
4 large tomatoes, coarsely chopped
6 large sprigs each mint and parsley, roughly chopped
1 cup blueberries
1/2 quantity standard French dressing (see page 132)

1 Put the bulgur wheat into a bowl, cover with cold water, and leave until swollen—about 30 minutes.

2 Drain the bulgur. Mix in the cucumber, onion, tomatoes, mint, and parsley. Sprinkle with the blueberries, pour on the dressing, and serve.

ORAC value per serving ★★

kiwi fruit, berries, and cottage cheese

Contrary to popular perception, the kiwi fruit is not just a decorative addition to your cooking. In fact, it's extremely rich in vitamin C—far more per 4 ounces than oranges—and is also a good source of fiber, beta-carotene, and vitamin E. In this dish, the unusual combination of strawberries and balsamic vinegar results in a surprising and interesting flavor, enhanced by the high ORAC scores of the blueberries and green bell pepper.

4 large kiwi fruit, peeled and sliced widthwise
8 large strawberries, sliced lengthwise
1 large green bell pepper, seeded and finely cubed
1 1/2 cups cottage cheese
Coarsely ground black pepper
1 cup blueberries
6 large sprigs mint, finely chopped
1/2 cup extra-virgin olive oil
2 tablespoons organic balsamic vinegar
1 teaspoon Dijon mustard

1 Arrange the kiwi fruit and strawberries alternately around the rims of four small plates.

2 Mix the green bell pepper with the cottage cheese and season well with coarsely ground black pepper.

3 Put a mound of the cottage cheese mixture in the middle of each plate and sprinkle with the blueberries.

4 Sprinkle the mint over the blueberries.

5 Mix the oil, vinegar, and mustard together and pour over the cottage cheese.

ORAC value per serving ★★★★

watercress, Belgian endive, and alfalfa

Like all sprouted seeds, alfalfa sprouts are a rich source of nutrients, designed by nature to provide everything the growing plant needs. With all the cancer-protective chemicals in watercress, the natural sugars in grapes, and plenty of vitamin C, this is a maximum-vitality dish with an enormous ORAC score.

About 8 cups watercress
3 heads Belgian endive
1 large, sweet Spanish onion, finely chopped
2 1/4 cups seedless black grapes, halved
9 cups alfalfa sprouts (or 5 cups bean sprouts), washed and drained
1 quantity creamy yogurt dressing (see page 133)

1 Wash and pick over the watercress and separate the Belgian endive heads into separate leaves.

2 Place the watercress and Belgian endive in a bowl, add the onion, grapes, and alfalfa (or bean) sprouts, and mix.

3 Pour on the dressing, mix again, and serve.

ORAC value per serving ★★★

red, red, red

Trust the French to come up with the idea of eating radishes smeared with butter and dipped in coarse sea salt—delicious, but hardly a treat for your heart and blood pressure. Here, the fabulous health properties of the radish, which, together with garlic and onions, was used by the ancient pharaohs to pay the workers building the pyramids, gives the bite to this high-ORAC salad.

1 large head radicchio
1 large red bell pepper, seeded and finely diced
1 1/2 cups sliced radishes
4 small, cooked beets, diced
1 small red onion, finely sliced
1 cup cranberries
1 quantity creamy yogurt dressing (see page 133)
10 young sprigs chervil

1 Arrange a nest of radicchio leaves in a large bowl.

2 Mix together the red bell pepper, radishes, beets, and onion and put into the radicchio nest.

3 Mix the cranberries gently into the dressing and pour over the salad.

4 Serve sprinkled with the whole chervil sprigs.

ORAC value per serving ★★

sweet and peppery

Mixing the sweetness of raspberries and watermelon with the hot peppery taste of watercress and the mild flavor of red onion is what gives this salad its unique "fusion" appeal. I first ate watercress and onion as a salad in a beach café overlooking the Indian Ocean on the island of Mauritius, where, strangely, watercress is the favorite salad ingredient.

About 4 cups watercress
1/2 watermelon, seeded and cut into bite-size cubes
1 large red onion, very finely chopped
2 cups raspberries
1 cup organic, unfiltered apple juice
Coarsely ground black pepper

1 Pick over the watercress and put into a salad bowl. Add the watermelon and onion and mix.

2 Sprinkle with the raspberries.

3 Pour on the apple juice and top with lots of coarsely ground black pepper.

ORAC value per serving ★★

green and red fusilli

Like all pasta salads, this one is substantial enough to be a meal on its own. Energy-giving carbohydrates, protein, calcium, masses of beta-carotene, and cholesterol-lowering monounsaturated fat from the olive oil also make this extremely healthy, with an excellent ORAC score.

4¹/₄ cups mixed tomato and spinach fusilli
Florets of 1 large head broccoli, very large ones halved
3³/₄ cups baby spinach
1 red onion, very finely chopped
1¹/₄ cups seedless black grapes, halved
¹/₂ cup extra-virgin olive oil
3 tablespoons freshly grated Parmesan cheese

1 Cook the pasta according to the package instructions. Drain and put into a large, warm bowl.

2 Meanwhile, plunge the broccoli into a saucepan of rapidly boiling water for 5 minutes.

3 Wash the spinach, leaving any water still clinging to the leaves. Place in another pan, cover, and cook until wilted—this should take 3–5 minutes, depending on the age of the leaves.

4 Drain the green vegetables and tip them into the pasta with the onion and grapes. Stir gently but thoroughly, being careful not to break up the broccoli florets.

5 Pour the olive oil over the mixture, add the Parmesan, mix gently again, and serve.

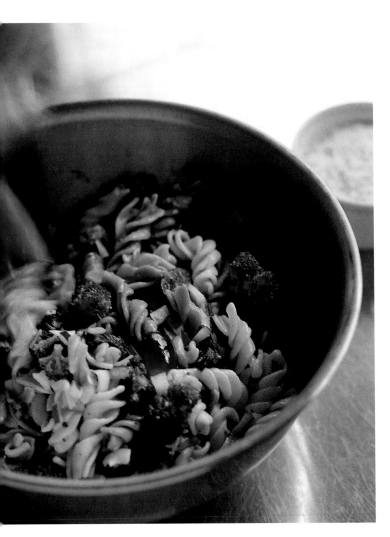

ORAC value per serving ★★

beans bonus

All beans are a healthy addition to the diet, as they contain protein, carbohydrates, vitamins, minerals, and fiber, with the bonus of phytoestrogens. It's these natural plant hormones that are so important for women, as they help prevent osteoporosis and control the unpleasant side effects of menopause. Combining fava beans and chickpeas with all the other ingredients provides a generous helping of essential nutrients and a high ORAC score.

3 cups shelled baby fava beans—frozen are fine if you can't find fresh
1 1/3 cups canned or cooked chickpeas, rinsed and drained
2/3 cup sun-dried tomatoes, snipped into slivers
3 large scallions, finely chopped
1 bulb fennel, trimmed and sliced lengthwise
Leaves of 3 sprigs fresh thyme
3 stalks sage, finely chopped
4 stalks Italian parsley, finely chopped
4 large plum tomatoes, coarsely chopped
1 quantity creamy yogurt dressing (see page 133)

1 Cook the fava beans and pinch them to remove the skins. This isn't strictly necessary and it is rather time-consuming, but it does make a difference to both the look and flavor of the dish.

2 Put the beans into a large salad bowl. Add the chickpeas, sun-dried tomatoes, scallions, fennel, thyme, sage, parsley, and fresh tomatoes and mix thoroughly.

3 Pour on the salad dressing, mix again, and serve.

ORAC value per serving ★★★

Mediterranean mix

Here's another recipe redolent of hot summer days and balmy evenings on the beach anywhere in the Mediterranean. Wonderful ripe tomatoes, succulent and flavorsome sweet peppers, and the coolness of cucumber add up to a feast of vitamins and a superprotective antiaging ORAC score.

1 1/2 cups frozen corn
1 red bell pepper, seeded and finely diced
1 yellow bell pepper, seeded and finely diced
1 cucumber, peeled, seeded, and diced
1 1/4 cups sliced radishes
1 sweet Spanish onion, finely chopped
5 plum tomatoes, finely chopped and juices retained
2/3 cup raisins
1 quantity standard French dressing (see page 132)

1 Cook the corn and leave to cool.

2 Put into a bowl with the peppers, cucumber, radishes, onion, tomatoes, and raisins.

3 Pour the dressing on top, mix gently, and serve.

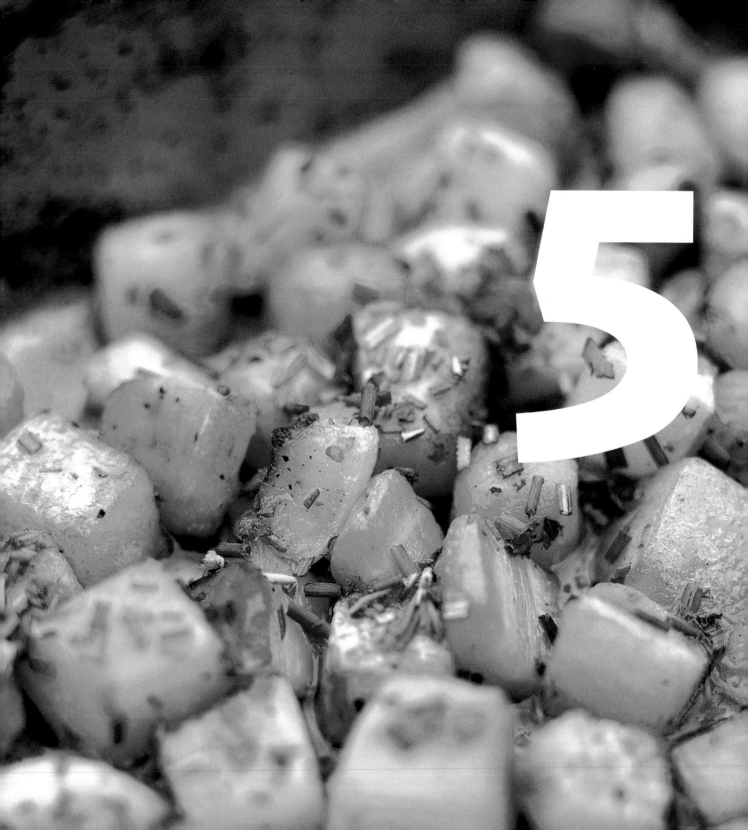

5

light meals

All recipes in this chapter serve 4 unless otherwise stated

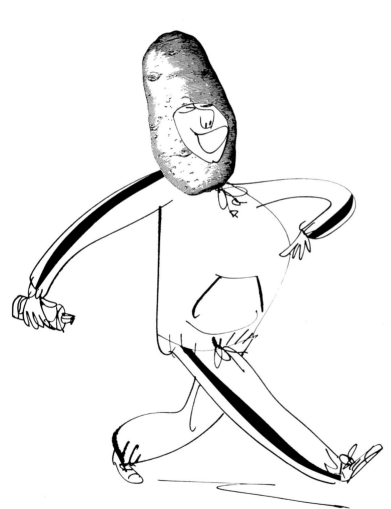

ORAC value per serving ★★

Spanish omelet

Equally good to eat hot or cold, this is a satisfying and substantial light meal. It's extremely rich in vitamin C and has lots of good carbohydrates, iron, B vitamins, and protein from the eggs, and all the protective natural chemicals from the onion.

3 cups frozen peas
5 tablespoons olive oil
1 cup peeled and diced potatoes
1 large onion, roughly chopped
2 red bell peppers, seeded and cubed
Salt and pepper
12 free-range organic eggs, well beaten

1 Place the peas in a saucepan of water, boil for 3 minutes, then drain.

2 Heat the oil in a very large skillet, or two small ones (if you're cooking in batches, divide the ingredient amounts between the pans).

3 Add the potatoes and stir until just turning golden.

4 Add the onion and peppers and cook until soft.

5 Stir in the peas.

6 Season the eggs, pour into the pan, and leave until the edges start to firm. Gently tip the pan to distribute the eggs evenly. When the base is firm but the top still runny, put under a hot broiler to finish cooking.

ORAC value per serving ★★★

broccoli, cauliflower, and cheese

Either a light meal for four or an excellent vegetable dish with a main course, comfortably serving six to eight people. The cancer-protective properties of broccoli and cauliflower are well documented, and the lycopene from the dried and fresh tomatoes adds a huge prostate-protective boost for men and helps reduce the risk of breast cancer for women.

1 large cauliflower, separated into florets
2 large heads broccoli, separated into florets
1 cup canned sun-dried tomatoes, drained and halved
1/4 cup unsalted butter
2 tablespoons flour
3 cups 2% milk
11/4 cups grated strong cheddar cheese
4 large plum tomatoes, sliced
2 tablespoons freshly grated Parmesan cheese

1 Preheat the oven to 425°F. Place the cauliflower and broccoli florets into a pan of boiling water. Cook for 5 minutes, drain, and rinse under cold water.

2 Arrange alternate florets in rows in a flat casserole dish and sprinkle with the sun-dried tomatoes.

3 Heat the butter gently in a large skillet. When melted, stir in the flour and cook for 2 minutes, stirring constantly, until the mixture thickens.

4 Gradually add the milk, again stirring continuously, and continue cooking until it forms a sauce. Add the grated cheese and stir until it's completely melted. Pour the sauce over the vegetables and arrange the plum tomatoes on top.

5 Sprinkle with the Parmesan, place in the oven, and bake for 20 minutes, until the sauce is bubbling.

ORAC value per serving ★★★

vegetable risotto

Don't even think about risotto if you haven't got arborio rice, as no other variety works as well. The combination of peas, asparagus, and baby spinach is what gives this creamy, light risotto such a good ORAC score, with the bonus of extra calcium from the mascarpone.

3 tablespoons olive oil
4 plump scallions, cut into large chunks
11/4 cups arborio rice
11/4 cups frozen peas
12 asparagus tips
4 cups basic stock (see page 30)
3 cups baby spinach or arugula
3 tablespoons mascarpone cheese

1 Heat the oil in a large saucepan, add the scallions, and sauté gently for 2 minutes. Add the rice and stir for 1 minute.

2 Mix in the peas and asparagus tips and add enough stock just to cover. Stir until the stock is almost absorbed. Continue gradually adding stock and stirring gently, without breaking up the asparagus tips, until the rice is tender.

3 Add the spinach or arugula and stir for 1 minute. Remove from the heat, stir in the mascarpone cheese, and serve.

ORAC value per serving ★ ★ ★

guacamole and salad

I've never understood why most people—and especially women—worry about avocados being fattening. They avoid them like the plague, put sweeteners and skim milk in their coffee, and then eat a Danish pastry! Avocados contain monounsaturated fats, which are heart-protective and help the body get rid of cholesterol. They're also extremely rich in vitamin E, which is known to protect against some forms of cancer and helps prevent heart and circulatory diseases. This delicious light meal has an extremely high ORAC score.

2 large ripe avocados
1/4 cup lemon juice
2 garlic cloves, finely chopped
2 large tomatoes, chopped
5 tablespoons plain organic yogurt
1 teaspoon Worcestershire sauce
2 large tomatoes, sliced
1 large red onion, sliced
6 cups alfalfa sprouts
1 quantity standard French dressing (see page 132)
8 whole-wheat pita breads

1 Peel the avocados and mash them roughly.

2 Put into a bowl with the lemon juice, garlic, chopped tomatoes, yogurt, and Worcestershire sauce and mix thoroughly. Refrigerate.

3 Place the tomato slices, onion, and alfalfa sprouts in a salad bowl, pour on the dressing, and mix.

4 Warm the pita bread, cut each one in quarters, and serve with the guacamole dip and salad.

ORAC value per serving ★ ★

pickled herrings with potato and tomato salad

A variation of the popular Scandinavian dish, this one adds to the essential oil and vitamin D in the herrings a huge amount of lycopene and a good ORAC score from the tomatoes. If you can't find pickled herrings, it is easy to pickle your own, but do it at least five days in advance.

12 ounces new potatoes
4 pickled herrings
1 1/3 cups sun-dried tomatoes, cubed
1/4 cup extra-virgin olive oil

If using fresh herrings:
1 large onion, sliced
1 large dill pickle
30 whole black peppercorns
Enough milk to cover the herrings
1 cup white wine vinegar

1 If using fresh herrings, remove the heads and tails. Gut and soak in cold water for 12 hours, then in milk for 12 hours. Slice each one down the center and remove the bones. Divide half the onion and dill pickle between the fillets, add six peppercorns to each, roll them up individually, and secure with toothpicks. Place in a large glass jar. Fill the jar with boiled vinegar, add the remaining sliced onion, dill pickle, and peppercorns, and secure the lid. Leave for at least 4 days.

2 Scrub the potatoes but don't peel them. Place in a saucepan of water, bring to a boil, and cook until just tender. Leave to cool slightly.

3 Quarter the potatoes and mix with the tomatoes. Drizzle with the olive oil. Place each herring on a plate and serve with the potato and tomato mixture on the side.

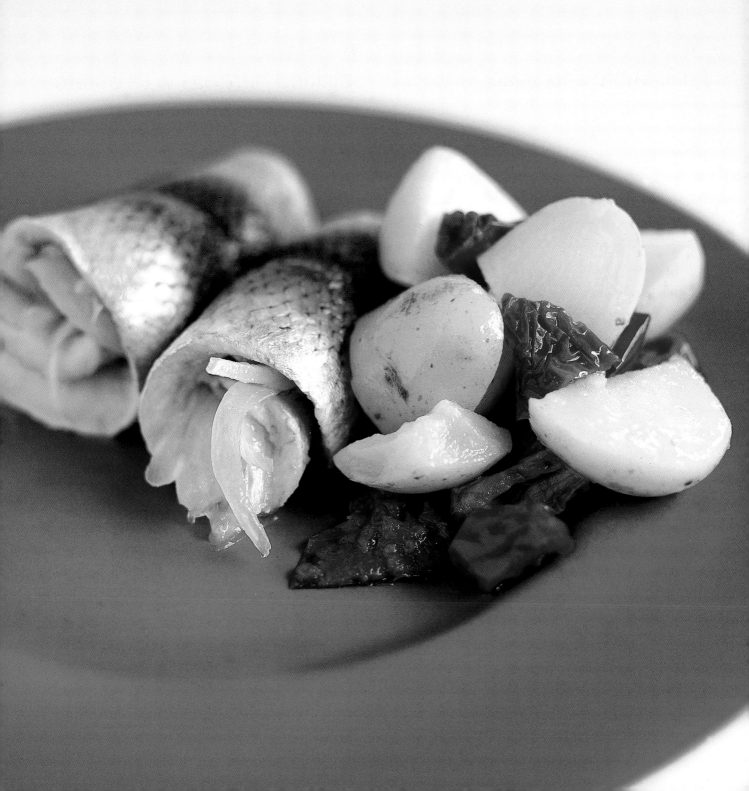

ORAC value per serving ★★★
stuffed red peppers

Wonderful to eat hot or cold, but I love them just warm in the Italian style. Red peppers are a nutritional feast on their own, and when you add the valuable antioxidants in corn and the unique lung-cancer protective chemicals in watercress, you have an ORAC feast as well.

2/3 cup rice
2 tablespoons extra-virgin olive oil
1 large onion, finely chopped
1 cup frozen corn
About 2 1/2 cups watercress, stems removed
4 large red bell peppers—choose squat vegetables with flat
    bottoms, as they have to stand up during cooking
8 tablespoons freshly grated Parmesan cheese
1 quantity hot tomato salsa (see page 123)

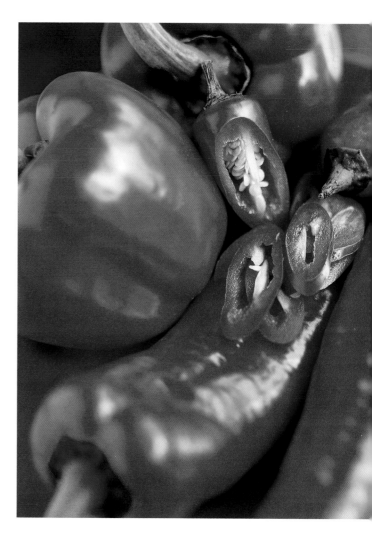

1 Preheat the oven to 350°F.

2 Cook the rice according to instructions on the package.

3 Heat the oil in a deep skillet or saucepan, add the onion, and sauté gently until soft—about 5 minutes.

4 Drain the cooked rice, pour into the onion, and stir until coated with the oil. Add the corn and mix thoroughly.

5 Add the watercress leaves and mix again.

6 Cut the peppers in half widthwise, trim the stalk until that end can sit upright, and remove the seeds and thick membrane. Soak the peppers in boiling water for 5 minutes.

7 Drain and stand the halved peppers in a large baking or casserole dish and spoon the rice mixture into each cavity. Add 5 tablespoons of water to the dish, cover with foil, and bake for 30 minutes.

8 Remove the foil, sprinkle on the Parmesan cheese, and bake for 10 minutes.

9 Serve with the hot tomato salsa on the side.

ORAC value per serving ★★⤝
vegetable stir-fry

Epidemiologists—scientists who study the health of different populations—have long known about the health benefits of the way people eat in the Far East. There, the most common cooking utensil is the wok, and stir-frying is one of the best ways of conserving the nutrient content of vegetables, cooking them very quickly and maintaining their color and flavor. This is real fast food, with a healthy ORAC bonus.

3 tablespoons canola oil, preferably organic
3 carrots, cut into 1 inch julienne strips
3/4 cup fine green beans, trimmed and halved
1 cup frozen corn, thawed
3 heads bok choy, trimmed, cut into sixths lengthwise, woody
*   parts removed*
3 1/2 cups alfalfa sprouts and 2 cups bean sprouts—if you can't
*   find alfalfa, use 4 cups bean sprouts*
1 quantity fresh tomato sauce (see page 122)
2 tablespoons light soy sauce

1 Heat the oil in a wok or very large skillet, tip in the carrots and beans, and stir-fry for 2 minutes.

2 Add the corn and bok choy and continue to stir-fry for 1 minute or until the bok choy is just wilted.

3 Add the alfalfa and bean sprouts and cook for 1–2 minutes, until cooked but still crunchy.

4 Pour in the tomato sauce and soy sauce, reduce heat slightly, and stir until heated through—about 3 minutes.

ORAC value per serving ★★⤝
tofu and honey treat

In parts of the world where soy-based foods are eaten regularly there's only a fraction of the osteoporosis that we suffer in the West, and women going through menopause are spared most of the unpleasant symptoms, especially the hot flashes. The reason is that those women eat far more natural plant estrogens, which are here in abundance, thanks to the tofu. Adding the monounsaturated oil and minerals in walnuts, with the benefits of beans, cranberries, and garlic, makes this a tasty and crunchy light meal.

1 garlic clove, finely chopped
1 tablespoon honey
1 teaspoon hot pepper sauce
1 tablespoon light soy sauce
1 1/4 cups diced tofu
1 1/2 cups green beans, or 2 1/3 cups snow peas or sugar snap peas
1/2 cup fresh or frozen cranberries, thawed
3 tablespoons canola oil
3/4 cup chopped walnuts

1 Mix together the garlic, honey, hot pepper, and soy sauce. Pour over the tofu and place in the refrigerator for 1 hour.

2 Meanwhile, cook the beans or peas—about 15 minutes.

3 If you haven't had time to thaw the frozen cranberries, leave them for 10 minutes in enough boiling water just to cover.

4 Heat the oil in a large skillet. Add the cranberries, walnuts, and drained tofu and cook gently, stirring constantly, for 2 minutes. Add the tofu marinade, mix in the beans or peas, and heat through.

ORAC value per serving

tuna and bean salad

As well as having a good ORAC score, this quick and simple dish provides essential fatty acids and vitamin D from the tuna, lots of essential vitamins and minerals, and a huge amount of soluble fiber to help control cholesterol and improve digestion.

4 free-range organic eggs
1¹/4 cups canned kidney beans, rinsed and drained
1¹/4 cups canned cranberry beans, rinsed and drained
1¹/4 cups canned flageolet beans, rinsed and drained
1 cup canned corn, rinsed and drained
2 cups drained canned tuna (preferably in spring water)
1 large red onion, chopped
2 large carrots, shredded
1 red bell pepper, seeded and cubed
3 large handfuls arugula (or baby spinach), thick stems removed
6 tablespoons standard French dressing (see page 132)

1 Semi hard-boil the eggs: put into cold water, bring to a simmer, and cook for 6 minutes. Peel the eggs and cut into quarters.

2 Put the drained beans, corn, and tuna into a large bowl. Mix in the onion, carrots, pepper, and arugula. Pour on the dressing and toss the salad to mix.

3 Serve with the eggs on top.

ORAC value per serving

corn, sweet potato, and beet fritters

These fritters can be eaten hot or cold with a salad as a light meal, but they also make an excellent accompaniment floating on top of soups or used as a base on which to serve other dishes. The horseradish and beet sauce adds an unusual hot, sweet flavor as well as boosting the ORAC score.

1 cup frozen corn, thawed
2 large sweet potatoes, peeled and grated
4 beets, cooked (but not pickled) and grated
2 tablespoons flour
2 free-range organic eggs, beaten
Canola oil, for frying
Horseradish and beet sauce (see page 125)

1 Mix the corn, potatoes, and beets together in a bowl.

2 Whisk the flour into the eggs and mix into the vegetables.

3 Form the vegetable mixture into eight equal portions and flatten.

4 Pour enough oil into a skillet to cover it to a depth of about ¹/4 inch. Fry the fritters for about 3 minutes on each side.

5 Serve with horseradish and beet sauce and a green salad.

ORAC value per serving ★★★⸜

tofu and noodle stir-fry

Superhealthy though it may be, even its most dedicated fans would have to admit that tofu equals tasteless. Happily, it's great at absorbing flavors, and marinating it in this fantastic mixture of lime, mango, hot pepper sauce, and garlic results in a piquant taste. This is a very high ORAC dish, with the bonus of containing one of the most cancer-protective of all the cabbage family—kale.

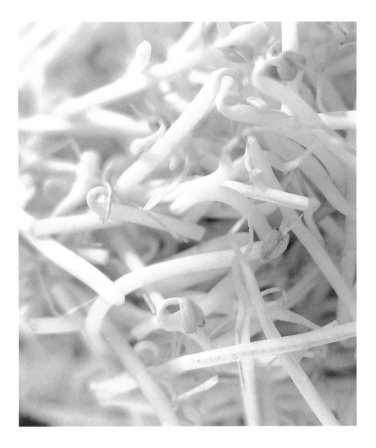

2 tablespoons lime juice
1 large mango, peeled, pitted, and chopped
1/2 teaspoon hot pepper sauce
2 garlic cloves, finely chopped
1 1/4 cups tofu, cubed
1/4 cup sesame oil
1 onion, chopped
1 cup instant egg noodles or rice noodles
4 cups finely shredded kale
5 1/2 cups alfalfa sprouts or 3 1/4 cups bean sprouts

1 Preheat the oven to 425°F.

2 Mix the lime juice, mango, hot pepper sauce, and half the garlic in a large ovenproof dish. Add the tofu, stir to coat in the marinade, and set aside for 30 minutes.

3 Place the tofu in its marinade in the oven and bake for 20 minutes.

4 Meanwhile, heat the oil in a wok or large skillet. Add the onion and remaining garlic and soften for 5 minutes.

5 In a saucepan, cook the noodles according to package instructions—usually around 2 minutes.

6 Add the kale to the onions and garlic and cook, stirring continuously, until wilted.

7 Still stirring, add the alfalfa sprouts and cook until transparent.

8 Drain the noodles, add to the vegetables, and cook for an additional 2 minutes.

9 Remove the tofu from the oven, add to the vegetables with the marinade, stir, and serve.

ORAC value per serving ★★

sardine and tomato pâté with watercress salad

There's no doubt that, generally speaking, fresh food is best. But there are three exceptions—canned sardines being one. (Tomatoes and beans also: tomatoes for their higher lycopene content, and beans for their convenience.) Superior to any bought fish pâté, this dish has bone-building calcium and vitamin D, lung-protective watercress, and a good ORAC score.

8 ounces canned sardines, drained
3 tablespoons tomato paste
1 tablespoon horseradish sauce (see page 124)
5 tablespoons unsalted butter
8 plum tomatoes, halved lengthwise
8 scallions, trimmed and shredded lengthwise
About 2 1/2 cups watercress, woody stems removed
French dressing (mix together 3 tablespoons oil and 1 tablespoon vinegar; add salt and pepper to taste)

1 Mash the sardines and stir in the tomato paste and horseradish sauce.

2 Melt the butter, being careful not to burn it. Add half to the fish mixture and mix well.

3 Transfer the mixture to a terrine or other suitable container.

4 Push the plum tomatoes into the surface of the fish, cut side up, pour the rest of the butter over the top, and refrigerate for at least 1 hour.

5 Mix the scallions and watercress together in a bowl. Add the French dressing and toss.

6 Take the terrine from the refrigerator, slice, and serve with salad.

ORAC value per serving ★★

shrimp couscous with raisins

The mixture of couscous, raisins, and shrimp with the spicy fish dressing provides the distinctive Middle Eastern flavor of this recipe. Quick and simple, this makes a delicious light meal for four or an appetizer for six. You'll get beta-carotene, vitamins A and C, iron, and plenty of fiber, and you'll get a valuable ORAC score.

1 cup raisins
2 cups couscous
About 2 cups basic stock (see page 30)
1 cup cooked, peeled shrimp
1/2 large cucumber, peeled, seeded, and cubed
1 red bell pepper, seeded and cubed
1 green bell pepper, seeded and cubed
4 large plum tomatoes, seeded, peeled, and roughly chopped
4 scallions, finely chopped
1 large carrot, shredded
1 zucchini, peeled and shredded
Spicy dressing for fish salads (see page 133)

1 Put the raisins into freshly boiled water for 1 minute. Drain.

2 Add the raisins to the couscous and cook according to package instructions, using stock instead of water.

3 Add the shrimp and raw vegetables while the couscous is still hot. Pour on the dressing and stir to mix.

4 Serve while still warm, or cover with plastic wrap and leave in the refrigerator. Bring back to room temperature before serving.

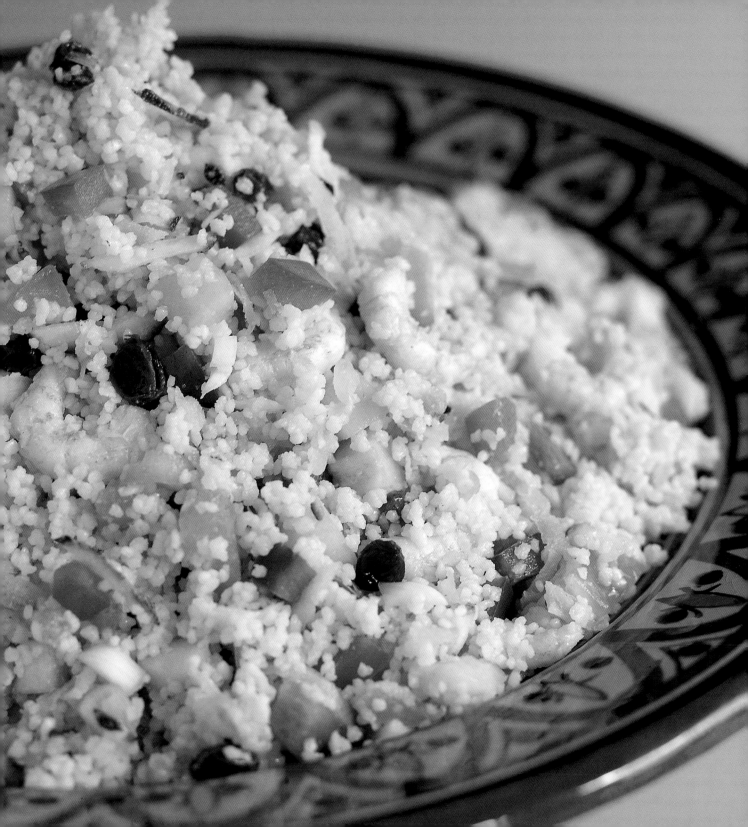

ORAC value per serving ★★

tuna fishcakes

Fishcakes are a perennial family favorite and taste just as good hot or cold. Two cakes is a substantial light meal, one makes an excellent appetizer. Oily fish like tuna is extremely heart- and skin-friendly because of the omega-3 fatty acids it contains. With the added nutritional value and cancer protection from the leafy green vegetables, you can turn a humble dish into a health fest.

7 ounces potatoes, peeled
10 ounces green leafy vegetables (kale, spring greens, cabbage, spinach, bok choy, etc.), shredded
1 1/2 cups drained canned tuna (preferably in spring water)
6 scallions, finely chopped
3 free-range organic eggs
6 tablespoons flour
Canola oil, for frying
1 head iceberg lettuce, shredded
1 quantity hot tomato salsa (see page 123)

1 Boil and roughly mash the potatoes.

2 Steam the green vegetables until tender—the timing will depend on the type of vegetables you're using.

3 Flake the tuna into a large bowl. Add the scallions, potatoes, and vegetables and mix thoroughly.

4 Beat the eggs in a bowl.

5 Tip the flour into another bowl.

6 With your hands, mold the fish and potato mixture into eight flat cakes. Dip each one first into the egg, then the flour.

7 Pour sufficient oil into a skillet to reach halfway up the fishcakes, and fry them, in batches, over a medium heat, until golden—about 5 minutes each side.

8 Drain the fried fishcakes on a double layer of paper towels.

9 Divide the lettuce between four plates and drizzle with some of the salsa.

10 Put the fishcakes on top and serve with the rest of the salsa on the side.

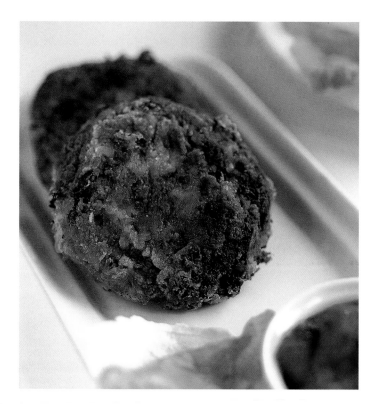

ORAC value per serving

macaroni and cheese

A favorite family standby that provides lots of calcium and protein, with the bonus of beta-carotene and minerals from the peppers and all of the heart and circulatory protection of garlic and onions. The addition of red peppers and parsley gives this far more eye appeal than ordinary macaroni and cheese, and the paprika spices up what can sometimes be a rather bland dish.

2 cups whole-wheat macaroni
2 tablespoons unsalted butter
1 large onion, finely chopped
3 garlic cloves, finely chopped
2 large red bell peppers, seeded and diced
1 teaspoon paprika
2²/₃ cups whole milk
2 cups grated mature cheddar cheese
2 tablespoons freshly grated Parmesan cheese
Parsley leaves, finely chopped
Freshly ground black pepper

1 Cook the macaroni according to package instructions. Drain and return to the rinsed pan.

2 Melt the butter in a skillet. Add the onion and garlic and soften for 5 minutes. Stir into the macaroni.

3 Mix in the peppers and paprika.

4 Add the milk and cook, stirring continuously, for 10 minutes.

5 Add the cheddar and Parmesan cheeses and stir until thoroughly mixed and the cheese has melted. Sprinkle with the parsley and season to taste with freshly ground black pepper.

ORAC value per serving ★↲

spinach snack-attack

I've known the fussiest of child eaters to eat these spinach snacks, and although the iron in this wonderful vegetable isn't well-absorbed, its antioxidant value and beta-carotene content make it one of the most valuable of green-leaf vegetables. Add the lycopene and vitamin C from the tomatoes, sustaining carbohydrates, B vitamins, and fiber from the bread, and you have a delicious light lunch or snack.

12 cups baby spinach
2 tablespoons unsalted butter
2 tablespoons extra-virgin olive oil
2 garlic cloves, finely chopped
²/₃ cup pine nuts
2 tablespoons lemon juice
4 tomatoes, sliced
4 large slices whole-wheat bread

1 Wash the spinach and put it into a pan with only the water clinging to it. Add the butter, cover tightly, put on a medium heat, and, shaking the pan occasionally, leave until wilted—this should take no longer than 5 minutes.

2 Meanwhile, heat the oil in a skillet and sauté the garlic and pine nuts gently until just turning golden. Add them to the cooked spinach with the lemon juice.

3 Place the tomato slices on the bread and top with the spinach mixture.

ORAC value per serving ★✦

Welsh rabbit with sautéed apples and blueberries

Here's another family favorite with a bonus. The simple addition of apples, blueberries, and onions not only results in a succulent, sweet-and-sour flavor, but adds vitamins, minerals, and fiber to this protein- and calcium-rich dish.

1/2 cup unsalted butter

4 large pippin apples, peeled, cored, and sliced

3/4 cup blueberries

1 cup grated cheddar cheese

1 large onion, finely grated

1 teaspoon dry mustard

3/4 cup stout

4 large slices whole-wheat bread

1 To make the fruit, melt half the butter in a large skillet.

2 Add the apples and cook on a medium heat until golden. Reduce the heat slightly, add the blueberries on one side of the pan, and continue cooking for 5 minutes, turning the blueberries gently.

3 To make the Welsh rabbit, put the cheese and onion into another pan with the mustard and stout. Stir until well combined and cook gently for 2 minutes.

4 Toast the bread on one side in the broiler. Turn over, pile on the cheese mixture, and broil for 5 minutes.

5 Place equal amounts of the apple and blueberry mixture on the side of four plates. Put the Welsh rabbit next to it and serve.

ORAC value per serving ★✦

stuffed celery and Belgian endive

Cottage cheese is very low in fat and calories, but the thought of eating one more portion brings a tear to the eye of anyone who has battled with weight-loss diets. Its boring texture and bland flavor don't make it food for the gourmet. But mix it with a hint of chives, the crunchiness of carrots, the sweetness of raisins, and the peppery flavor of cancer-protective watercress and alfalfa sprouts, finished with the iron-rich bitterness of Belgian endive, and it's food to titillate the most jaded palate.

2/3 cup seedless raisins

1 cup cottage cheese

2 carrots, shredded

12 chives, snipped

2 1/2 cups watercress, chopped

2 heads Belgian endive, separated into leaves

4 thick celery ribs, cut into 2 inch pieces

1/2 cup alfalfa sprouts

1 Soak the raisins in simmering water for 5 minutes. Drain and mix into the cottage cheese.

2 Add the carrot, chives, and watercress and mix again.

3 Arrange the Belgian endive leaves and celery on four plates.

4 Pile the cottage cheese mixture onto the Belgian endive leaves and celery.

5 Sprinkle with the alfalfa sprouts and serve.

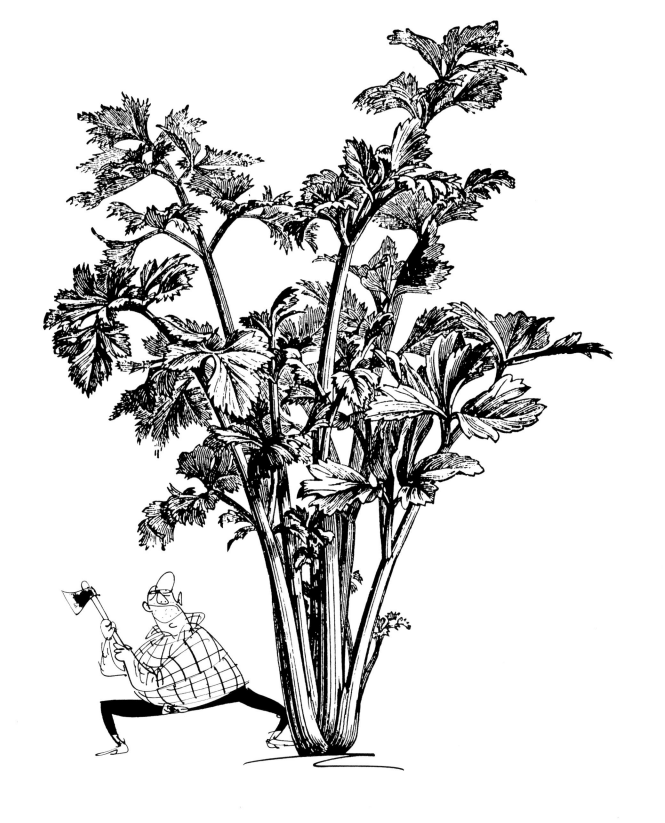

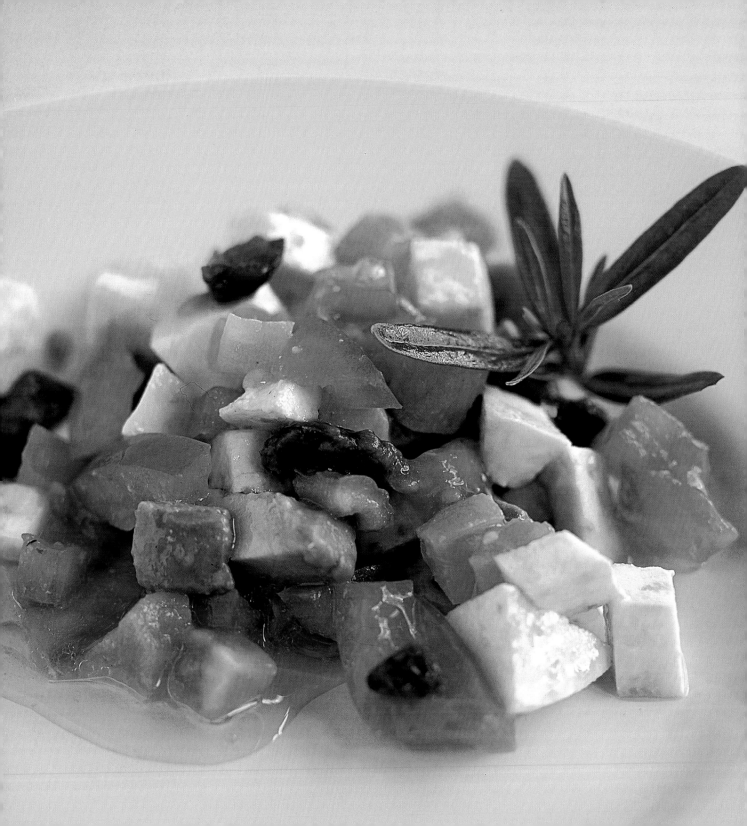

ORAC value per serving ★★

pasta with anchovy, garlic, and lemon sauce

An instant, no-cook sauce, with vitamin D and essential fatty acids from the anchovies, lycopene from the sun-dried and fresh tomatoes, bioflavonoids and vitamin C from the lemon, lots of carbohydrates from the pasta, and the cleansing benefits of parsley and chives.

12 ounces spaghettini
8 slices sun-dried tomatoes
2 tablespoons capers
1 1/4 cups canned anchovy fillets
2 garlic cloves, crushed
2 teaspoons grated lemon rind
3 tablespoons lemon juice
6 tablespoons extra-virgin olive oil
4 large, fresh tomatoes, roughly chopped
3 large sprigs parsley, chopped
12 chives, snipped

1 Cook the pasta according to package instructions. Meanwhile, soak the sun-dried tomatoes in freshly boiled water for 5 minutes. Drain, chop finely, and set aside.

3 Soak the capers in milk for 5 minutes, then drain.

4 Drain most of the oil off the anchovies. Put the fish into a mortar or mixing bowl, add the capers, garlic, and grated lemon rind, and crush with a pestle or fork.

5 As the mixture starts to break down, pour in the lemon juice. Add the olive oil gradually, stirring until the mixture forms a paste.

6 Add the paste to the drained pasta and mix well.

7 Stir in the drained sun-dried tomatoes and the fresh tomatoes, sprinkle with the parsley and chives, and serve.

ORAC value per serving ★★★★

tomato, mozzarella, and avocado salad

A far cry from the ubiquitous tricolore salad of Italian restaurants in the 1970s. Here, the slabs of red tomatoes, white mozzarella cheese, and green avocados are complemented by the hugely nutritious dried fruits, massive amounts of vitamin C from the kiwi fruit, and an extremely high ORAC score. A salad to turn back your biological clock.

1 cup mixed dried fruits (dates, pitted prunes, apricots,
*   raisins, etc.), cut into raisin-sized pieces*
2 quantities standard French dressing (see page 132)
2 1/2 cups drained and cubed young mozzarella cheese
4 large tomatoes, roughly chopped
2 avocados, peeled, pitted, and cubed

1 Soak all the fruits in freshly boiled water for 5 minutes. Drain thoroughly and stir into the dressing.

2 Put the mozzarella, tomatoes, and avocados into a large bowl.

3 Pour the fruit dressing over the top, mix well, and serve.

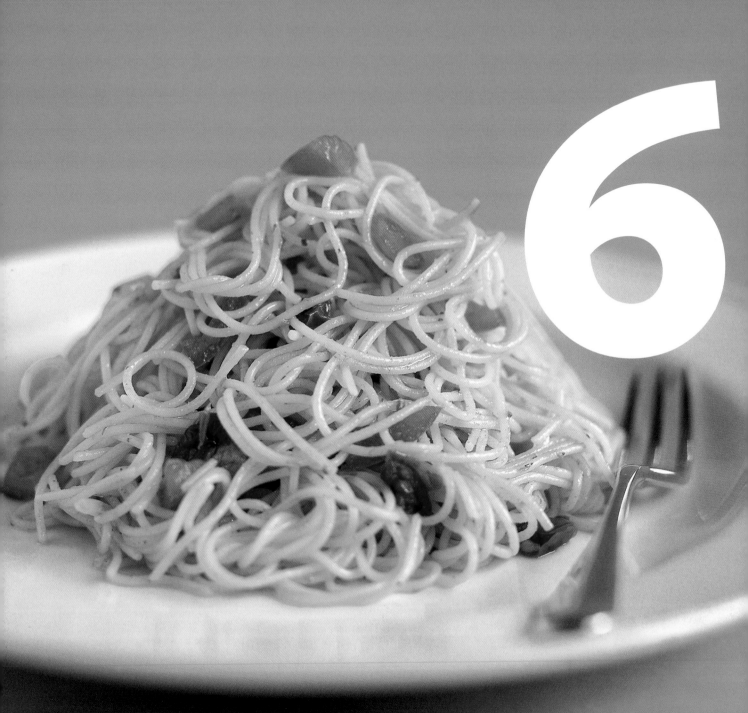

main

courses

All recipes in this chapter serve 4

ORAC value per serving ★✦

fusilli with tomato sauce

This vegetarian dish is a one-pot meal with a good ORAC score and an exceptionally high anticancer value thanks to the cabbage, kale, and leeks and the lycopene in the tomato sauce.

4¹/₄ cups basic stock (see page 30) or stock made with
 salt-free stock cubes
4¹/₄ cups tricolore fusilli
¹/₄ large Savoy cabbage, roughly chopped
2 large leeks, roughly chopped
4 large leaves kale, roughly chopped
1³/₄ cups fresh tomato sauce (see page 122)
1 large avocado

1 Bring the stock to a boil in a large saucepan.

2 Add the fusilli and chopped green vegetables and simmer until the pasta is just tender.

3 Meanwhile, heat the tomato sauce.

4 Peel, pit, and mash the avocado.

5 Remove the tomato sauce from the heat and mix in the avocado until blended.

6 Drain the pasta and vegetables and put into a large bowl. Serve with the tomato and avocado mixture on top.

ORAC value per serving ★★✦

Dutch Indonesian lamb

This warm lamb and salad is easy to cook and fun to eat, since you have to pick up the chops with your fingers.

1 small red bell pepper, seeded and roughly sliced
6 dried dates, quartered
2 tablespoons crunchy peanut butter
1 tablespoon tahini
1 teaspoon soy sauce
2 garlic cloves
Up to 5 tablespoons extra-virgin olive oil
2 racks of lamb, 6–8 chops each
About 4¹/₄ cups mixed green lettuce
1 quantity standard French dressing (see page 132)

1 Put the pepper, dates, peanut butter, tahini, soy sauce, and garlic into a blender and puree, adding olive oil as necessary to keep the mixture smooth.

2 Pull most of the thick fat off the lamb. Rub the mixture over the meat and refrigerate for about 1 hour to let the flavors combine.

3 Preheat the oven to its maximum temperature. Put the lamb in the oven with the peanut mixture still on top. Reduce the heat to 400°F and roast for 35 minutes.

4 Remove from the oven, cover loosely with foil, and let rest for 10 minutes.

5 Meanwhile, wash the lettuce and toss in the salad dressing.

6 Cut the racks of lamb into chops. Put the salad on a serving plate and arrange the lamb chops on top.

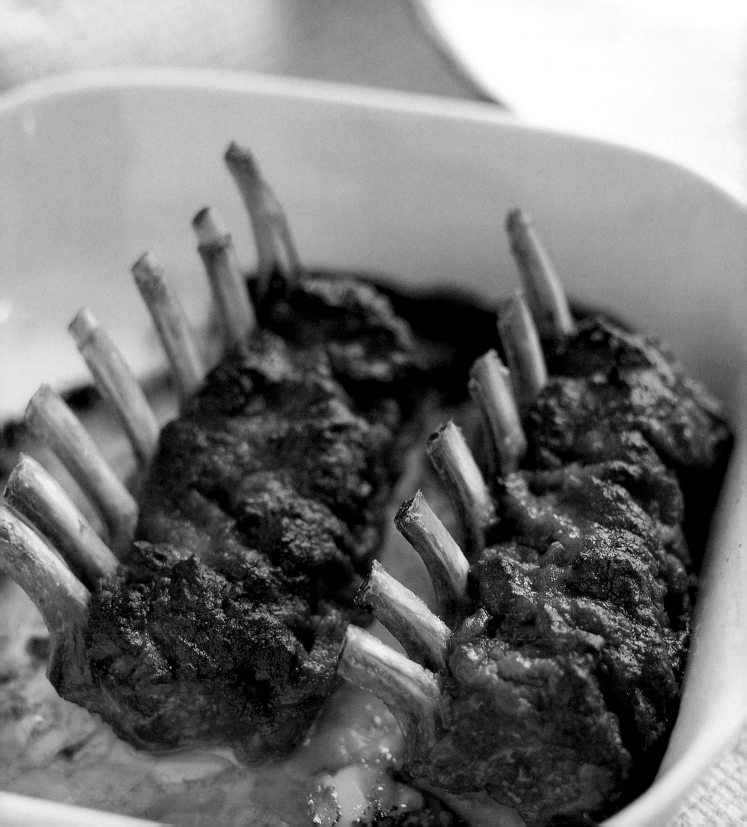

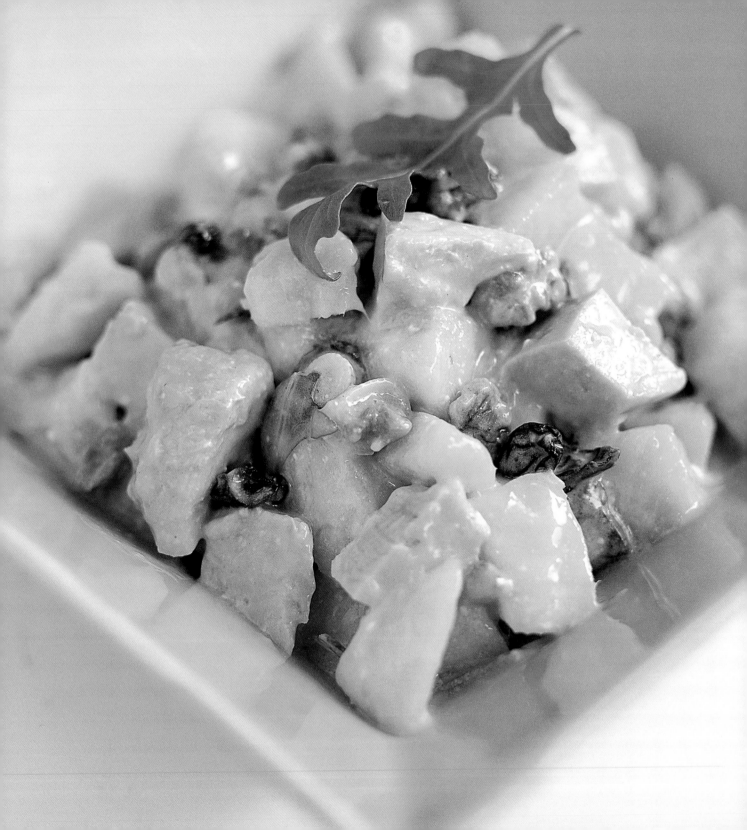

ORAC value per serving ★★⌡

mango chicken

More taste of the Pacific Rim as the exotic flavors of mango are combined with simple roast chicken. As well as the high ORAC value, the walnuts provide additional heart protection with their monounsaturated fats. The sweetness is offset by the bite of arugula.

1 small, cold cooked roast chicken
2 ripe mangoes, cubed
1/4 cup fresh lime juice
4 large scallions, finely sliced
2/3 cup raisins
1/2 cup extra-virgin olive oil
2 tablespoons organic mayonnaise
1/2 cup chopped walnuts
7 cups arugula, torn

1 Roughly chop the chicken; discard the skin and bones.

2 Mix the chicken, mangoes, lime juice, scallions, and raisins with the oil and mayonnaise.

3 Add the walnuts and arugula.

4 Stir all the ingredients together and serve.

ORAC value per serving ★

pasta arabiata

Sometimes called the devil's sauce because it can be devilishly hot—it's the chili that stimulates the circulation.

3 garlic cloves, chopped
Leaves of 3 sprigs fresh parsley
4 sprigs fresh oregano or marjoram, left whole
1 teaspoon chili powder
1/2 teaspoon cayenne pepper
1/4 cup extra-virgin olive oil
2 teaspoons red wine vinegar
2 tablespoons tomato paste
3 large, flat mushrooms
2 zucchini, cut into 1 inch slices
1 cup frozen corn
1 pound dried penne
3 tablespoons freshly grated Parmesan cheese

1 Put the garlic, parsley, oregano or marjoram, chili powder, cayenne pepper, olive oil, and vinegar into a blender and blend for 1 minute until smooth.

2 Add the tomato paste and 2 teaspoons of water, and blend for 3 seconds.

3 Add the mushrooms, zucchini, and corn to the blender and blend for 1 minute, adding water if the sauce looks too thick.

4 Cook the penne according to instructions on the package or until al dente. Drain.

5 Warm the puree over a low heat until it just begins to bubble. Stir it into the hot pasta and serve sprinkled with the Parmesan.

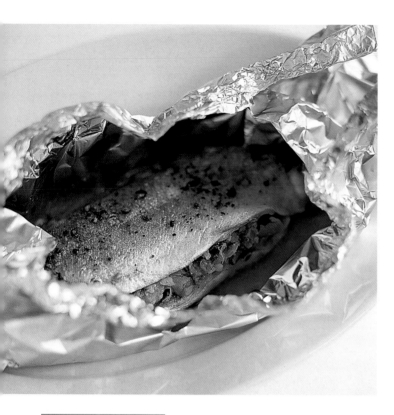

1¹/4 cups canned chickpeas, drained
4 large sprigs Italian parsley, finely chopped
3 tablespoons lemon juice
4 small sea trout, trimmed and cleaned
¹/2 cup dry white wine
¹/4 cup unsalted butter
Coarsely ground black pepper

1 Preheat the oven to 425°F.

2 Heat the oil in a skillet, add the onions and garlic, and sauté for 5 minutes.

3 Stir in the paprika and cayenne pepper and cook for an additional 2 minutes.

4 Add the tomatoes and chickpeas and simmer until tender—about 10 minutes.

5 Mash the mixture roughly, pouring off any excess tomato juice until you have the consistency of a stuffing.

6 Add the parsley and lemon juice and mix into the stuffing.

7 Pile the stuffing into the trout cavities.

8 Cut four pieces of foil big enough to totally envelop each fish. Put each trout on a piece of foil. Divide the wine among them, dot with the butter, season generously with coarsely ground black pepper, and seal the pockets.

9 Bake for 20 minutes. Open the foil carefully to let the steam escape before serving.

ORAC value per serving ★✈

baked stuffed trout

Trout has good nutritional value for the money and is easily available, but I think people get bored with having it just plain, steamed, broiled, or pan-fried with almonds. Try this interesting and extremely healthy recipe with distinct overtones of the Middle East.

¹/4 cup extra-virgin olive oil
1 small onion, finely chopped
1 garlic clove, finely chopped
1 teaspoon paprika
1 teaspoon cayenne pepper
1¹/3 cups canned chopped tomatoes

ORAC value per serving ★ ✔

California risotto

You can't make risotto in a hurry, but the whole ethos of "slow food" is the use of traditional methods to conserve flavor, texture, and nutrients. Cooking risotto is as therapeutic as any form of meditation and more relaxing than a bucketful of Prozac. The only side effect is the substantial health benefit of the high ORAC score.

1 tablespoon extra-virgin olive oil
2 garlic cloves, chopped
5 scallions, chopped
2 small red chilies, seeded and finely diced
1 small red pepper, seeded and finely diced
1 small yellow pepper, seeded and finely diced
1 cup arborio rice
1 tablespoon coriander powder
2 tablespoons cumin powder
About 3³/4 cups basic stock (see page 30)
1¹/3 cups pitted prunes, snipped into ¹/4 inch pieces
Leaves of 3 large sprigs parsley, chopped
Leaves of 3 large sprigs cilantro, chopped

1 Heat the oil gently in a deep skillet or saucepan, add the garlic, scallions, chilies, and peppers, and simmer until soft—about 10 minutes.

2 Mix in the rice and stir until coated with the oil.

3 Add the coriander and cumin and cook for 3 minutes, stirring continuously.

4 Add a ladleful of stock, stirring until the liquid is absorbed.

5 Add the prunes to the rice with the second ladleful of stock.

6 Continue adding stock, a ladleful at a time, for about 20 minutes, until the rice is tender but still has some bite.

7 Serve sprinkled with the chopped parsley and cilantro leaves.

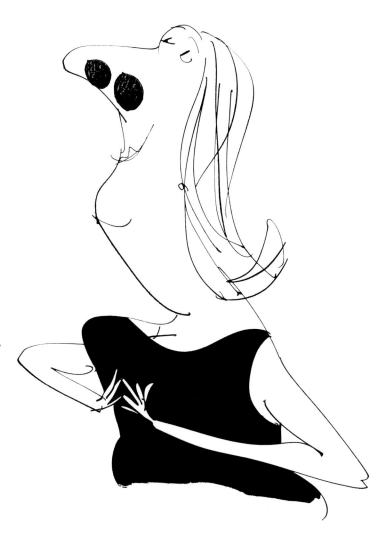

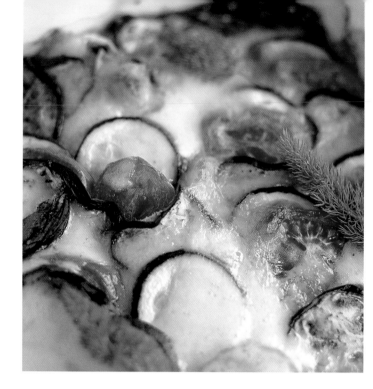

ORAC value per serving ★★

Sally's vegetarian sunshine bake

Here is the essence of the Mediterranean diet. It's not just the vitamins A, C, and E that you get from the oil and fresh vegetables, but the antioxidant properties in onions, garlic, eggplant, and tomatoes that make this such a protective dish. There's a bonus from calcium in the cheese and antibacterial essential oils in the oregano. Health benefits aside, this dish smells wonderful when it's cooking and it looks like a plate of sunshine.

6 tablespoons olive oil
3 sweet Spanish onions, diced
2 garlic cloves, finely chopped
3 large sprigs fresh oregano, roughly chopped. Dried oregano
*   won't be as good for aroma or flavor, but if you have to use it,*
*   add 1 tablespoon.*
2 small eggplants, cut into 1/4 inch slices
Salt
5 zucchini, peeled if necessary and cut into 1/4 inch slices
6 tomatoes, cut into 1/4 inch slices
1 pound fresh, young mozzarella cheese, cut into 1/4 inch slices
Freshly ground black pepper
5 tablespoons freshly grated Parmesan cheese
6 sprigs dill

1 Preheat the oven to 400°F.

2 Heat the oil in a skillet, add the onions, and cook gently for 5 minutes to soften.

3 Add the garlic and continue cooking for 3 minutes.

4 Stir the oregano into the onion mixture and remove from the heat.

5 Put the eggplant slices on a baking sheet in a single layer, sprinkle with salt, and bake for 8 minutes until softened.

6 Put the onion and herb mixture into an ovenproof dish. Arrange the eggplant, zucchini, tomato, and mozzarella alternately in the dish, standing them on their sides. When they're all arranged, push down gently with the palms of your hands and season with black pepper.

7 Place the dish in the oven and bake for about 1 hour.

8 Sprinkle with the Parmesan and bake for another 10 minutes.

9 Serve sprinkled with the whole sprigs of dill.

ORAC value per serving ★★★✦

vegetarian nutty bake

This is a nut roast with attitude. The combined nutritional value of the root vegetables, prunes, oats, and other ingredients makes this a health-plus recipe, which will be enjoyed as much by committed carnivores as it will be by vehement vegetarians. This is super-ORAC food.

6 tablespoons unsalted butter
1 onion, finely chopped
2 garlic cloves, finely chopped
2¹/₂ cups peeled and finely diced mixed root vegetables (carrots, turnips, potatoes, etc.)
1 leek, cut into ¹/₄ inch slices
2 zucchini, cubed
2¹/₂ cups sliced chestnut mushrooms
¹/₂ cup whole-wheat flour
1¹/₄ cups basic stock (see page 30)
¹/₄ cup tomato paste
¹/₂ cup pitted prunes, quartered
2 large sprigs curly parsley, finely chopped
Freshly ground black pepper
1 cup rolled oats
³/₄ cup crushed mixed nuts

1 Preheat the oven to 350°F.

2 Melt 4 tablespoons of the butter in a large skillet.

3 Gently sauté the onion and garlic in the butter until soft—about 5 minutes.

4 Add the root vegetables to the pan and continue cooking gently for an additional 10 minutes.

5 Add the leek, zucchini, and mushrooms to the pan and cook for 1 minute.

6 Stir in the flour and cook for 1 minute, stirring continuously.

7 Pour in the stock, tomato paste, and prunes and stir until thickened.

8 Add the parsley, season well with freshly ground black pepper, and pour the mixture into an ovenproof dish.

9 Rub the remaining butter into the oats and nuts, sprinkle on the dish, and bake for 30 minutes.

ORAC value per serving ★★★

duck breasts in onion and fruit sauce

This unusual way of cooking duck is extremely simple. It's a perfect dish if you're entertaining, as you can prepare it in advance and reheat it when you're ready. It provides excellent protein and a massively protective ORAC score thanks to the prunes and cranberries.

1 cup dried cranberries
4 duck breasts
¹/₄ cup olive oil
2 large Spanish onions, finely diced
2 tablespoons whole-wheat flour
1 cup orange juice
¹/₂ cup dry white wine
2 large sprigs fresh thyme, finely chopped
¹/₂ cup pitted prunes, cut into cranberry-sized pieces

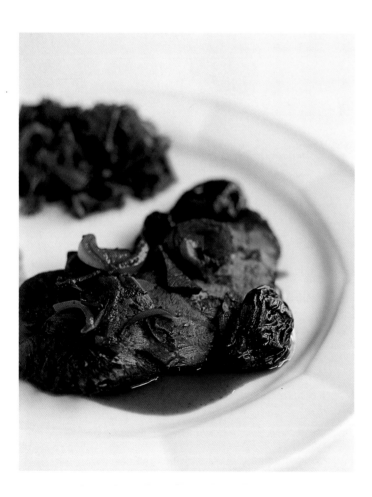

1 Pour enough boiling water over the cranberries just to cover them. Leave in a bowl.

2 Trim any fat off the duck breasts and flatten the breasts slightly with the back of a wooden spoon.

3 Heat half the oil in a large skillet and brown the duck breasts on both sides. Drain off the fat, transfer the meat to a warm plate, and reserve.

4 Clean the pan and heat the remaining oil in it. Add the onions and sauté gently for 5 minutes.

5 Add the flour and cook gently, stirring continuously, for an additional 2 minutes.

6 Drain the cranberries, reserving the liquid.

7 Keeping the pan on a low heat, gradually pour the orange juice, wine, and cranberry liquid into the onion and flour mixture.

8 Add the duck breasts, thyme, prunes, and cranberries. Cover and simmer for about 30 minutes, until the duck is tender.

ORAC value per serving ★★✈

chicken and prunes

The carrot, zucchini, and fresh herbs are all good sources of ORAC, but the addition of dried fruit and garlic makes this recipe the highly protective dish that it is—and also gives it a North African flavor.

4 skinless chicken breasts
¹/4 cup lemon juice
¹/4 cup extra-virgin olive oil
2 sprigs tarragon, left whole
4 bay leaves
2 large carrots, peeled and sliced
3 zucchini, sliced lengthwise
1 cup basic stock (see page 30) or chicken stock from the chicken soup recipe (see page 40)
6 pitted prunes
6 dried apricots
2 garlic cloves, finely chopped
³/4 cup fresh bread crumbs
2 tablespoons chopped fresh mixed herbs: tarragon, Italian parsley, chervil, and oregano

1 Flatten the chicken breasts with the back of a wooden spoon and put them into a deep ovenproof dish large enough to hold them in one layer. Cover with the lemon juice and 3 tablespoons of the oil.

2 Add the tarragon and bay leaves. Refrigerate for at least 1 hour, turning once. Remove the bay leaves.

3 Preheat the oven to 400°F.

4 Arrange the carrots and zucchini on the chicken, basting them with the marinade.

5 Add the stock, prunes, and apricots, cover with foil, and cook in the oven until tender—about 40 minutes.

6 Meanwhile, heat the remaining oil in a skillet and gently sauté the garlic.

7 Add the bread crumbs and stir until golden, then stir in the mixed herbs.

8 Sprinkle the chicken with the herb mixture and serve.

ORAC value per serving ★★★✦

trout with prune relish

Here's another interesting way to cook trout, which will also supply the majority of your day's ORAC needs for optimum protection. Making the prune relish is simple, and the finished dish has a wonderful richness. This prune relish goes equally well with other robust fish, game, rabbit, duck, goose, and ham.

1/4 cup lemon juice
2 sprigs cilantro, finely chopped
3 tablespoons olive oil
3 bay leaves
4 trout fillets
3 tablespoons unsalted butter
3/4 cup chopped mixed nuts
4 large scallions, chopped
2 garlic cloves, chopped
1/2 cup white wine vinegar, cider vinegar, or rice vinegar
3 plum tomatoes, chopped
15 pitted prunes, chopped

1 Mix half the lemon juice and half the cilantro with the oil. Add the bay leaves, pour over the trout, and refrigerate for 1 hour.

2 Remove the fish from the marinade and reserve the liquid.

3 Put the fish on a broiler pan, brush with the marinade, and broil for about 5 minutes each side, basting every minute or so.

4 Meanwhile, melt the butter in a skillet. Add the nuts and sauté for 2 minutes.

5 Add the scallions, garlic, vinegar, and the remaining lemon juice and cook gently for an additional 2 minutes.

6 Add the tomatoes and prunes with the rest of the cilantro and cook for an additional 2 minutes.

7 Serve the trout with the relish on top.

ORAC value per serving ★★

Persian beef stew

There has been a remarkable renaissance of traditional Persian cooking in the last few years. The cooking is healthy and the savory dishes are deliciously flavored with spices like cinnamon and nutmeg, more usually associated with desserts.

3/4 cup yellow split peas, rinsed
1 tablespoon extra-virgin olive oil
1 large onion, finely chopped
12 ounces lean stewing beef, trimmed of fat and cubed
1 teaspoon cinnamon
1/4 teaspoon grated nutmeg
2 2/3 cups basic stock (see page 30)
1 large cooking apple, peeled, cored, and thickly sliced
1 sweet potato, peeled and cubed
2 tablespoons lemon juice
2 tablespoons honey
1/2 cup raisins
1 cup frozen green peas
Salt and pepper

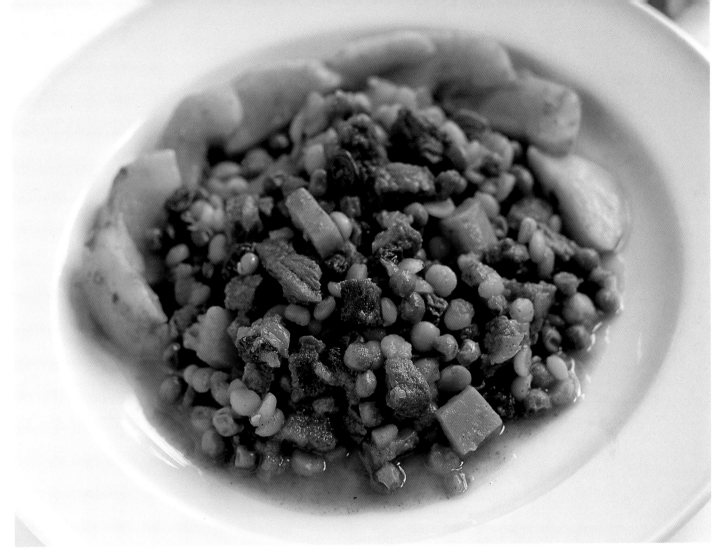

1 Put the split peas in a bowl, cover with water, and leave for 1 hour.

2 Heat the oil in a large, deep skillet, add the onion, and sauté for 3 minutes, until softened.

3 Add the meat and continue cooking, stirring continuously, until the meat is seared and the onion slightly golden.

4 Stir in the cinnamon and nutmeg, add the stock, and simmer, covered, for 30 minutes.

5 Drain and rinse the split peas. Put into a saucepan of boiling water and boil for 5 minutes. Drain.

6 Add the split peas to the pan with the apple and potato. Bring back to a boil, cover, and simmer for 15 minutes.

7 Add the lemon juice, honey, raisins, and green peas, pushing the raisins and the peas into the pan without breaking up the apple. Continue to simmer for 15–20 minutes.

8 Season with salt and pepper, if necessary, and serve.

ORAC value per serving

three-bean, eggplant, and tofu casserole

It really isn't necessary to salt and press eggplant before you cook it—which I think puts people off from using this wonderful, high-ORAC vegetable. Tofu is another food that makes people turn up their noses, but as well as having a useful ORAC rating, it's about the best source of natural plant hormones, which have special protective benefits of their own. The delicious flavors of sesame, coconut, and cilantro make this dish well worth a try, so put aside your prejudices and be prepared for a pleasant surprise.

2 tablespoons extra-virgin olive oil
2 tablespoons unsalted butter
1 red onion, chopped
2 garlic cloves, chopped
1/2 teaspoon chili powder
2 teaspoons sesame seeds
1/2 large eggplant, peeled and diced
3/4 cup green beans, cut into 1 inch pieces
3/4 cup fava beans
11/4 cups canned kidney beans, rinsed and drained
Handful of chopped cilantro
11/4 cups cubed tofu
13/4 cups coconut milk
13/4 cups basic stock (see page 30)

1 Preheat the oven to 400°F.

2 Heat the oil and butter in a skillet and soften the onion and garlic in it for about 5 minutes.

3 Add the chili powder and sesame seeds and continue cooking for 1 minute.

4 Add the eggplant and cook for 2 minutes.

5 Transfer the contents of the pan to a casserole dish and add the green beans, fava beans, kidney beans, cilantro, and tofu.

6 Pour on the coconut milk and stock, adding more stock if necessary to cover the ingredients.

7 Bake for 40 minutes, checking occasionally to ensure the casserole isn't drying out.

ORAC value per serving

calf's liver with almonds

Although not exceptionally high in ORAC value, this is one of my favorite ways of cooking liver. Although organic calf's liver is expensive, it's worth every penny for its lack of unwanted toxic chemicals and its fabulous flavor. It also supplies masses of vitamins A and B12 and iron.

Leaves of 1 large sprig rosemary, finely chopped
2 garlic cloves, very finely chopped
2 cups fresh whole-wheat bread crumbs
11/4 cups ground almonds
2 pinches ground saffron
1/4 cup extra-virgin olive oil
Freshly ground black pepper
1/4 cup unsalted butter
4 slices calf's liver, about 6 ounces each
1/2 cup red wine

1/2 cup raisins
Steamed carrots and broccoli, to serve

1 Mix the rosemary, garlic, bread crumbs, almonds, and saffron into half the oil. Season with black pepper.

2 Heat the butter and remaining oil in a large skillet. Add the liver and cook for 3–4 minutes, depending on thickness and how pink you like it, turning once. Remove and keep warm.

3 Put all the other ingredients into the pan and boil briskly for 2 minutes, stirring to loosen any liver stuck to the bottom.

4 Serve the liver with the sauce spooned over the top and accompanied by steamed carrots and broccoli.

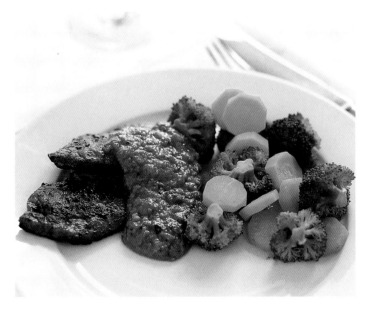

ORAC value per serving ★★★

curried bean and root vegetable stew

This is a perfect autumn or winter dish, and it's ideal for a slow cooker. Get it ready the night before, turn on the slow cooker before you go to work, and when you return, you'll be greeted by mouthwatering smells and a meal bursting with ORAC to protect against winter chills and ills.

3 tablespoons canola oil—ideally organic
1 large leek, sliced
1 large onion, chopped
3 garlic cloves, finely chopped
3 teaspoons curry powder or paste
1 rutabaga, cubed
1 large parsnip, cubed
2 carrots, cubed
1 sweet potato, peeled and cubed
About 3 cups basic stock (see page 30)
2 1/3 cups canned organic crushed tomatoes
3 tablespoons tomato puree
2 1/2 cups canned fava beans, rinsed and drained

1 Heat the oil in a large saucepan and sauté the leek, onion, and garlic, stirring continuously, for 3 minutes.

2 Add the curry powder or paste, stir until it coats the vegetables, and cook for an additional 2 minutes. Add the root vegetables to the pan and stir to coat thoroughly. Add the stock, crushed tomatoes, and tomato puree, and bring to a boil. Cover and simmer for 45 minutes.

3 Add the fava beans and continue to simmer until the beans and all the other vegetable are tender—about 10–15 minutes.

ORAC value per serving ★★★★★★★★

braised duck with prunes

Here's a recipe that's a poke in the nose for all those food police who try to persuade everyone that healthy eating should be the culinary equivalent of sackcloth and ashes. The combined flavors of duck, shallots, Armagnac, and prunes are worthy of any top-class restaurant, but the recipe is simplicity itself. It's full of protein; has the heart-protective benefits of garlic, shallots, and red wine; has lots of fiber from the dried fruit; and you'll get huge amounts of beta-carotene. Add a simple salad for vitamin C and you'll have everything your body needs—with an extraordinarily high ORAC score.

2 tablespoons extra-virgin olive oil

4 duck breasts

²/₃ cup bacon cubes

7 shallots, quartered

3 tablespoons Armagnac

2 tablespoons flour

2²/₃ cups red wine

10 pitted prunes

10 dried apricots

3 garlic cloves, finely chopped

1 bouquet garni

1 Preheat the oven to 425°F.

2 Heat the oil in a skillet and brown the duck breasts on both sides. Remove and keep warm.

3 Brown the bacon and shallots in the pan.

4 Return the duck to the pan, pour in the Armagnac, and set alight. When the flames die down completely, stir in the flour and mix thoroughly.

5 Transfer the contents of the pan to a casserole dish.

6 Add half the wine to the skillet, with the prunes, apricots, garlic, and bouquet garni. Bring to a boil, then add to the casserole dish. Pour in the rest of the wine and bake for 20 minutes.

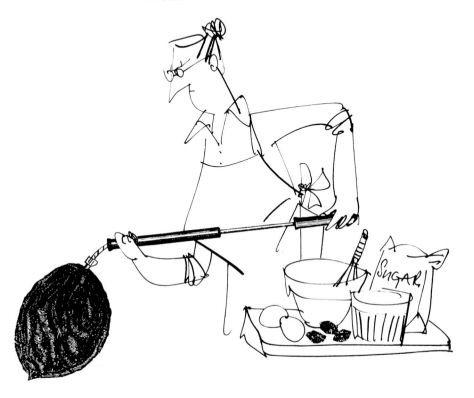

ORAC value per serving ★★✈

New Orleans herb gumbo

This is a very traditional Creole vegetarian gumbo, redolent of the hot, steamy swamplands and the flavors of allspice and cloves. This style of New Orleans cooking was born out of poverty and, like all peasant food, it's nourishing, filling, and sustaining. It's also exceptionally protective.

3/4 cup whole-wheat flour
6 garlic cloves
2 tablespoons extra-virgin olive oil
1 large onion, chopped
1 red bell pepper, seeded and cubed
2 large celery ribs, sliced
2 pinches allspice powder
1 cup long-grain rice
3 pounds mixed green leafy vegetables (spinach, spring greens, cabbage, kale, chard, Brussels sprouts, etc.)
3 bay leaves
1 teaspoon dried basil
1 teaspoon dried thyme
2 pinches ground cloves
Salt and pepper to taste
Leaves of 1 large sprig curly parsley, chopped
2 pinches cayenne pepper
1 teaspoon soy sauce
2²/3 cups hot tomato salsa (see page 123)

1 Brown the flour by heating gently in a dry skillet, stirring constantly. Remove and reserve.

2 Finely chop three of the garlic cloves.

3 Heat the oil in a saucepan, add the chopped garlic, onion, pepper, and celery, and sauté until soft—about 5 minutes.

4 Add the browned flour and allspice, stir well, and set aside.

5 In a separate saucepan, cook the rice according to package instructions.

6 Mash the remaining garlic cloves.

7 In another pan, cook all the vegetables in just enough water to cover, with the mashed garlic, bay leaves, basil, thyme, and ground cloves, for 5 minutes.

8 Drain, reserving the cooking liquid, and chop, removing the bay leaves and any large pieces of garlic.

9 Gradually add about 15 ounces of the vegetable water to the flour mixture, adding extra water if necessary to make up the quantity. Stir constantly over a low heat until completely smooth.

10 Pour the mixture over the vegetables and stir thoroughly. Season with salt and pepper, mix in the parsley, cayenne pepper, and soy sauce thoroughly.

11 Drain the rice and pour the vegetable mixture on top. Serve with the hot tomato salsa on the side.

ORAC value per serving ★★⌐

ham and kidney bean gumbo

Another great gumbo from the Louisiana bayous, which typifies the culinary melting pot of the Choctaw Indians, the Cajuns, the French, and the awful heritage of the African slave trade. Tradition tells us that this recipe was referred to as "washday gumbo," served on Monday, when the women were too busy with the washing to spend hours cooking. It was prepared when they had time on Sunday and, like so many stews, tasted even better the following day. This recipe is extremely rich in a wide variety of nutrients.

1¼ cups brown rice
2 tablespoons sunflower oil
1 red onion, chopped
2 garlic cloves, chopped
1 celery rib, sliced
1 small green bell pepper, seeded and cubed
1 small red bell pepper, seeded and cubed
1½ cups finely cubed lean ham
3 cups canned kidney beans, rinsed and drained
½ teaspoon dried thyme
½ teaspoon dried oregano
6½ cups basic stock (see page 30)
1 tablespoon soy sauce
1 teaspoon hot pepper sauce

1 Cook the rice according to package instructions. If it's done before the gumbo is ready, drain, cover, and keep warm.

2 Heat the oil in a large saucepan and sauté the onion and garlic gently until softened.

3 Add the celery and peppers and continue sautéing gently for 4 minutes.

4 Add the ham and continue to sauté for an additional 4 minutes.

5 Mix in the beans, herbs, stock, soy sauce, and hot pepper sauce, and simmer until the beans are tender—5–10 minutes.

6 Drain the rice and serve the gumbo on top.

ORAC value per serving ⌐

veggie honey-roast tofu

Not a very high ORAC recipe, but extremely rich in soy isoflavones—plant hormones that are especially protective for women against breast cancer, osteoporosis, and the discomforts of menopause. It also has a good level of fiber from the root vegetables and a healthy balance of omega-3 and omega-6 fatty acids from the canola oil. Boost the ORAC rating with any of the sauces or compotes in chapter 9.

¼ cup canola oil—ideally organic
3 tablespoons honey
3 tablespoons light soy sauce
1 parsnip, cut into bite-size cubes
1 sweet potato, peeled and cut into bite-size cubes
1 large red apple, peeled, cored, and cut into bite-size cubes
1¼ cups cubed tofu
Freshly ground black pepper

1 Preheat the oven to 375°F.

2 Brush a baking tray with some of the oil.

3 Put the rest of the oil in a small saucepan and melt the honey in it over a low heat. Add the soy sauce.

4 Put the vegetables and apple into a bowl, pour in half the soy sauce mixture, and stir to coat thoroughly.

5 Transfer to the baking tray, cover with foil, and put in the oven to roast, stirring occasionally.

6 Meanwhile, put the tofu in the rest of the sauce, making up an extra quantity if needed and adding three twists of fresh, coarsely ground black pepper. Leave to marinate.

7 After 40 minutes, add the tofu to the baking tray and return to the oven, uncovered, for another 20 minutes.

ORAC value per serving ★★✦

gvetch: Romanian one-pot vegetable stew

Another truly peasant recipe, named after the gvetch pot in which it is cooked. Made without meat—an expensive luxury for agricultural workers—this wonderful mixture of fresh and dried beans and green and root vegetables provides protein for growth, carbohydrates for energy, and plenty of vitamins and minerals. It's also a high-ORAC dish.

1 small sweet onion, chopped
2 garlic cloves, chopped
1 small white potato, peeled and sliced
1 small sweet potato, peeled and sliced
1/4 small green cabbage, such as Savoy, coarsely chopped
3/4 cup button mushrooms, halved
1 bay leaf
1 small carrot, cut into 1 inch pieces
1/2 celery rib, cut into 1 inch pieces
1 small green bell pepper, seeded and diced
1 head broccoli, cut into florets
1/2 eggplant, sliced
11/2 cups canned lima beans, rinsed and drained
Leaves of 2 large sprigs Italian parsley, chopped
1/3 cup fresh green beans, sliced into thirds
1 tomato, thinly sliced
11/4 cups tomato juice
Salt and pepper

1 In a narrow, deep saucepan, layer all the ingredients from onion to green beans in the order they appear in the list above.

2 Arrange the tomato slices on top.

3 Pour in the tomato juice.

4 Cover the pan and bring slowly to a simmer. Cook, tightly covered, for about 30 minutes, adding water if the mixture seems to be drying out.

5 Leave to rest for 15 minutes, then add salt and pepper to taste.

ORAC value per serving ★★

fish risotto

This is one of our family favorites for a light, nourishing, late dinner on Fridays after a long and busy week. Sally has this recipe down to a T. The delicious, crunchy texture of the snow peas, with the softness of the rice and fish, blends perfectly with the Asian flavor of curry. Excellent nutrition and a good ORAC recipe, too.

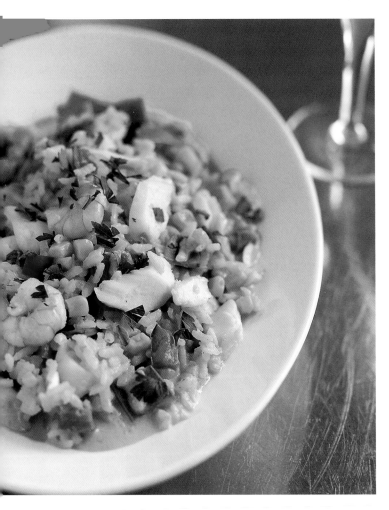

2 tablespoons canola oil—preferably organic

1 onion, chopped

1 garlic clove, finely chopped

2 teaspoons curry powder

1 small red bell pepper, seeded and diced

1 1/4 cups arborio rice

2 cups basic stock (see page 30)

2 cups coconut milk

12 ounces cod fillet or other firm fish such as hake, halibut, monkfish, haddock, fresh tuna, or swordfish—or 8 ounces fish and 1/2 cup cooked peeled shrimp

1 cup very young snow peas, cut into 1/2 inch lengths

1 cup canned corn, rinsed and drained

Leaves of 6 sprigs Italian parsley, coarsely chopped

1 Heat the oil in a deep skillet or saucepan and gently sauté the onion and garlic until soft—about 5 minutes.

2 Stir in the curry powder, mix thoroughly, and cook for 2 minutes.

3 Add the red pepper, rice, stock, and coconut milk and simmer for 20 minutes, until the rice is tender and nearly all the liquid has been absorbed.

4 Break the fish into bite-size chunks, stir into the rice mixture, mix well, and put back on a gentle heat for 5 minutes, adding more stock if the risotto looks as if it's drying out. Check that the firm fish is cooked—fish with denser flesh, such as monkfish and tuna, may take a few minutes longer.

5 Add the snow peas, corn, and shrimp (if using), and heat through for 2 minutes. Serve the risotto sprinkled with the parsley.

ORAC value per serving ★★✔

steamed fish in foil

A truly easy way to cook fish and the healthiest way to cook the vegetables, this produces a finished dish that is extremely high in essential nutrients and has a simple, clean flavor. The impressive ORAC score is a bonus.

4 steaks of salmon, halibut, or hake
2 small carrots, thinly sliced lengthwise with a vegetable peeler
1 orange bell pepper, seeded and cut into very fine strips
4 scallions, sliced lengthwise into strands
2 tablespoons lemon juice
1/2 cup dry white wine
1/4 cup unsalted butter
4 sprigs dill
Freshly ground black pepper
11/2 pounds mixed green leafy vegetables (spinach, chard, cabbage, kale, etc.), coarsely chopped
2 leeks, very finely sliced

1 Preheat the oven to 400°F.

2 Cut four pieces of foil large enough to envelop each piece of fish comfortably. Put each fish steak into the middle of a piece of foil. Add the carrots, pepper, and scallions.

3 Pull up the sides of the foil and pour in the lemon juice and wine. Dot each fish with butter, lay the dill on top, add a twist of freshly ground black pepper, and seal the pockets.

4 Bake in the oven for 20 minutes.

5 Meanwhile, put the green leafy vegetables into a steamer and cook until they're just tender but with bite—about 10 minutes.

6 When the fish is done, pile the green vegetables on individual serving plates. Carefully open one end of each pocket and pour the juices over the green vegetables. To serve, use a fish lifter or spatula to lift the fish, with the vegetables on top, onto the green vegetables.

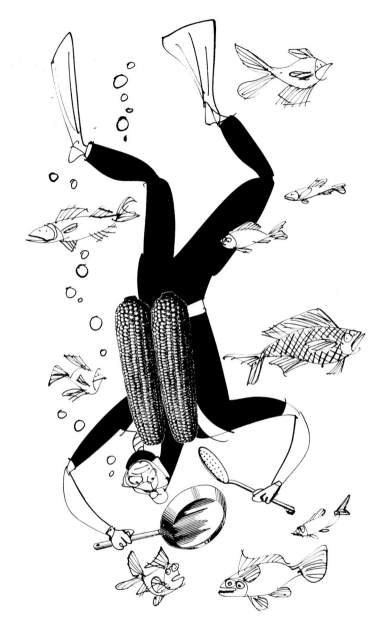

ORAC value per serving ★★

beef and couscous pilaf

Distinct flavors of North Africa enhance this substantial dish. The unique combination of pistachio nuts, beef, and spices is what produces the taste, but it's the addition of the peas and dried fruits that bump up the ORAC score. Including generous amounts of fresh mint improves digestion and offsets any fattiness in the beef.

Scant 1/2 teaspoon cumin
Scant 1/2 teaspoon cinnamon
1 teaspoon coriander
1/2 pound lean braising steak, cut into small cubes
2 tablespoons canola oil—preferably organic
1 1/2 cups couscous
1/2 cup dried apricots, each cut into six pieces
1/2 cup golden raisins
3 cups basic stock (see page 30)
3/4 cup shelled pistachio nuts
1 cup frozen peas
Leaves of 4 large sprigs mint, chopped

1 Mix the cumin and cinnamon and half the coriander.

2 Coat the meat with the spice mixture and set aside.

3 Heat half the oil in a large skillet, pour in the couscous, and cook, stirring continuously, for 2 minutes. Remove from the heat and stir in the remaining coriander.

4 Add the apricots to the couscous with the golden raisins.

5 Boil the stock and add half to the couscous, stir, cover, and leave to stand for 10 minutes.

6 Meanwhile, dry-fry the nuts gently for 5 minutes.

7 Fluff up the couscous with a fork and add the rest of the stock.

8 Cook the peas in boiling water for 2 minutes, sprinkle them on the couscous, cover, and set aside.

9 Heat the remaining oil in another pan, sear the steak, reduce the heat slightly, and continue cooking for 8 minutes or until as well done as you like it, stirring continuously.

10 Add the meat and nuts to the couscous and stir thoroughly.

11 Sprinkle with the mint and serve.

ORAC value per serving ★★★✔

stir-fried vegetables with shrimp

Like the French paradox and the Mediterranean diet, the way people eat in the Far East holds the secret of their good health. In this part of the world, fewer women have breast cancer, hardly any have osteoporosis, and there's not even a word for menopausal hot flashes. Heart disease, high blood pressure, and bowel cancer are also comparatively rare. It's not just that the people eat less meat, but much less fat, and burgers are, thankfully, still not part of their culinary culture. It's what they do eat that counts—and this great dish is a typical example.

1 tablespoon light soy sauce

1 tablespoon sherry vinegar

1/2 teaspoon hot pepper sauce

1 tablespoon sesame oil

1 teaspoon honey

2 tablespoons canola oil—preferably organic

2 carrots, finely sliced

11/2 cups sliced oyster mushrooms

1 head broccoli, cut into florets

2 heads bok choy, cut into eighths lengthwise

1/2 inch fresh ginger, peeled and grated

5 large scallions, quartered lengthwise

2 cups snow peas, cut into 3/4 inch pieces

8 raw king tiger shrimp in their shells

51/3 cups fresh bean sprouts

1/4 cup sesame seeds

1 Whisk together the soy sauce, sherry vinegar, hot pepper sauce, sesame oil, and honey and set aside.

2 Heat the canola oil in a wok or large, deep-sided skillet. Add the carrots, mushrooms, broccoli, bok choy, and ginger and cook, stirring continuously, for 3 minutes.

3 Add the scallions and snow peas and continue cooking for 1 minute.

4 Add the shrimp and cook for 4 minutes, until they start to change color.

5 Add the bean sprouts and cook for 1 minute.

6 Add the soy sauce mixture and 3 tablespoons water and cook gently until the vegetables are tender—about 4 minutes.

7 Meanwhile, dry-fry the sesame seeds in a separate pan.

8 Serve the stir-fry sprinkled with the sesame seeds.

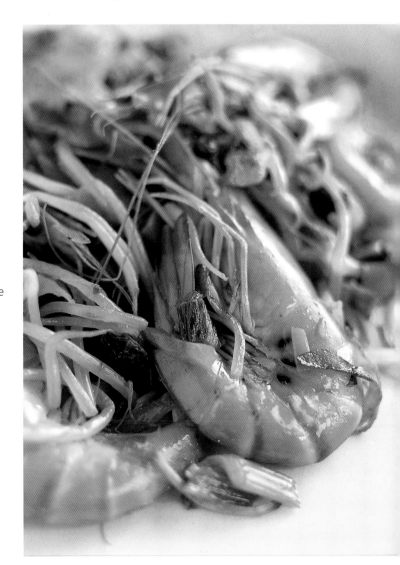

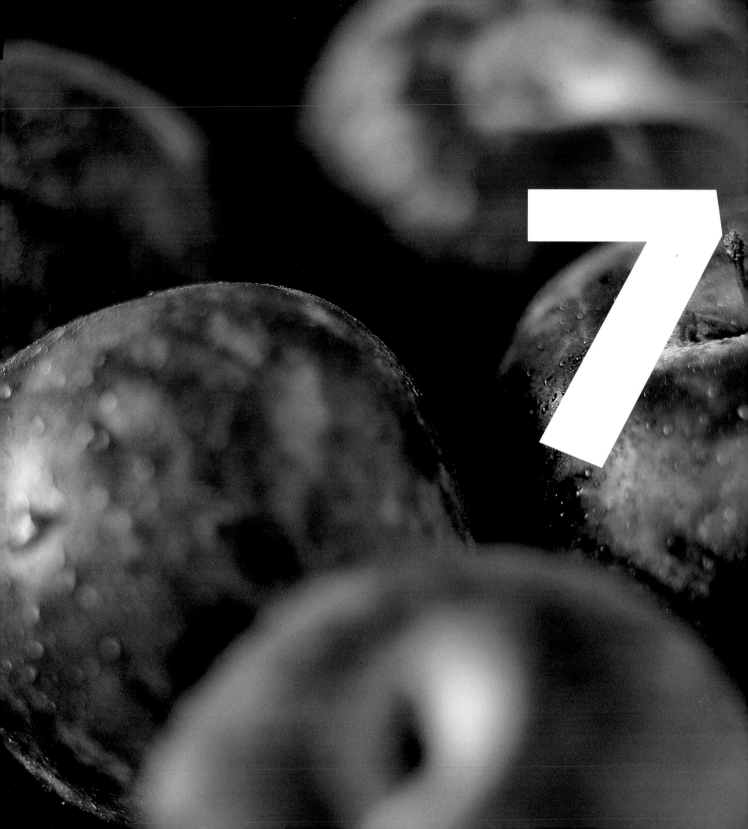

sweet
things

All recipes in this chapter serve 4

ORAC value per serving ★★★★★

fruity rice pudding

Rice pudding may sound like children's food, but this one has a sophisticated taste and a huge ORAC value. The traditional addition of nutmeg is a major feel-good factor, as this exotic spice is a great mood enhancer. This is a sweet thing and not remotely naughty.

1/3 cup long-grain rice
2 teaspoons brown sugar
2 2/3 cups milk
1 1/2 cups mixed dried fruits (prunes, apples, mangoes, apricots, raisins, cranberries, etc.), all cut to the size of raisins
3-inch cinnamon stick
1/2 teaspoon nutmeg
1/2 cup unsalted butter, chopped

1 Preheat the oven to 375°F.

2 Put the rice and sugar into an ovenproof bowl and add the milk and dried fruit.

3 Break the cinnamon stick in half and add to the bowl.

4 Sprinkle with the nutmeg and dot with butter.

5 Bake for 1 hour.

ORAC value per serving ★★

fruit gelatin

Not just a kids' favorite, but a highly protective, delicious treat—immensely rich in vitamin C, light and refreshing, so it's perfect after beef stews, roasts, or casseroles. Apart from its ORAC value, the vitamin C will make sure you get maximum absorption of iron.

2 tablespoons lemon juice
2 tablespoons honey
1 1/3 cups red grape juice
1 envelope gelatin powder, unflavored
2/3 cup red currants
1 cup strawberries, hulled and halved
3/4 cup raspberries
3/4 cup blueberries

1 Mix the lemon juice with the honey and grape juice.

2 Sprinkle the gelatin onto 1/4 cup of hot water (or per package instructions) and stir briskly until it swells.

3 Line a 6-cup loaf pan with plastic wrap.

4 Strip the fruit off most of the red currant stems, leaving one or two whole for decoration. Arrange in the loaf pan with the other fruit.

5 Heat the gelatin mixture gently until it dissolves, then stir into the grape juice mixture and pour over the fruit.

6 Put into the refrigerator until set, 1–2 hours, depending on your refrigerator temperature.

7 Turn out and decorate with the reserved red currant stems.

ORAC value per serving ★★★★⟋

tea bread with raisins and prunes

The delicate flavor of bergamot oil in the tea, the almost negligible fat content from the egg, and the enormous protective benefits of its ORAC score make this a treat you can enjoy without a single pang of guilt.

5 Earl Grey tea bags
1¹/₃ cups boiling water
1 free-range organic egg, beaten
1¹/₃ cups raisins
1¹/₄ cups prunes, cut to the size of raisins
1 cup brown sugar
2¹/₄ cups organic self-rising flour

1 Soak the tea bags in the water and leave until cold. Squeeze the tea bags and discard.

2 Mix all the ingredients together and leave on the counter for at least 6 hours.

3 Preheat the oven to 350°F.

4 Line a 6-cup loaf pan neatly with parchment paper. Spoon in the mixture and bake for 30 minutes or until a skewer inserted into the center comes out clean.

ORAC value per serving ★★★★

tea bread with dried cherries, cranberries, and apricots

The bite of ginger and the tanginess of the lemon and cranberries make this another fabulous tea bread, which you can enjoy on its own or as a dessert served with your favorite ice cream or yogurt sauce (see page 126).

5 lemon-ginger tea bags
1¹/₃ cups boiling water
2 cups mixed dried cherries, cranberries, and apricots
1 free-range organic egg, beaten
1 cup brown sugar
2¹/₄ cups organic self-rising flour

1 Soak the tea bags in the water and leave until cold. Squeeze the tea bags and discard.

2 Quarter the apricots.

3 Mix all the ingredients together and leave on the counter for at least 6 hours.

4 Preheat the oven to 350°F.

5 Line a 6-cup loaf pan neatly with parchment paper. Spoon in the mixture and bake for 30 minutes or until a skewer inserted into the center comes out clean.

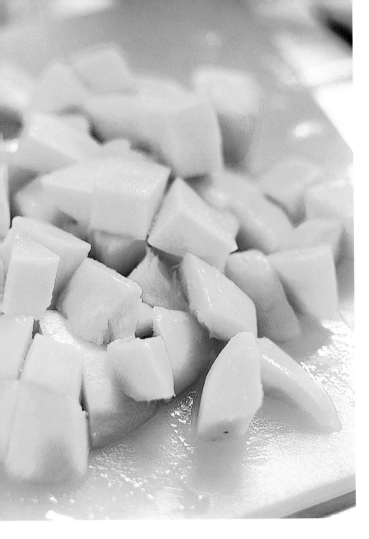

1 cup elderflower pressé or diluted elderflower cordial
$1/2$ cup sugar—but see directions below before adding all of it
2 cups cubed mangoes
2 cups red currants, stripped from stems
2 tablespoons lemon juice

1 Put the elderflower pressé or cordial into a saucepan. If the liquid you're using is unsweetened, add all the sugar. If it already has added sugar, use half the amount.

2 Bring slowly to a boil and boil for 4 minutes. Remove from the heat and leave to cool.

3 Meanwhile, mix together the mangoes and red currants. Puree and press through a medium strainer.

4 Combine the fruit with the elderflower liquid and lemon juice.

5 If you have an ice-cream maker that also makes sorbets, process according to instructions. If not, pour the mixture into a flattish freezerproof dish, place in the freezer, and leave until almost frozen.

6 Remove from the freezer and break up thoroughly with a fork or puree in a food processor. Return to the freezer and repeat the process.

7 Leave in the freezer until you have the texture you require; some people like sorbets more solid than others. If yours overfreezes, transfer to the refrigerator 2 hours before serving.

ORAC value per serving

mango and red currant sorbet

The delicate taste of elderflower, the succulent sweetness of the mango, and the acidity of fresh red currants combine to give this sorbet its unique flavor. It's an excellent source of beta-carotene, vitamin C, and ORAC.

ORAC value per serving ★★

passion fruit and blackberry sorbet

Although it's widely used in other parts of the world, rose water seldom appears in our everyday recipes. What a shame! Its distinctive taste and perfume enhance this unusual sorbet, which contains large amounts of vitamins C and E as well as having a high ORAC score.

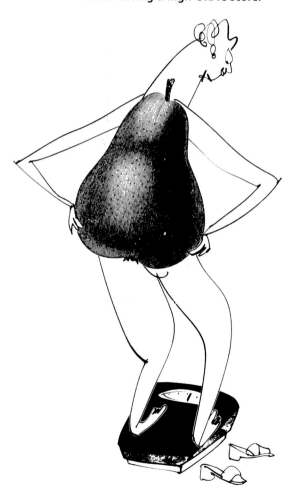

^{1}/$_2$ cup pink grapefruit juice
^{2}/$_3$ cup rose water
^{1}/$_2$ cup sugar
6 passion fruit
About 2^1/$_2$ cups blackberries

1 Mix the grapefruit juice and the rose water.

2 Put the mixture into a pan with the sugar, bring slowly to a boil, and boil for 4 minutes. Remove from the heat and leave to cool.

3 Meanwhile, scoop out the passion fruit and strain into a bowl, discarding the seeds.

4 Puree the blackberries, strain to remove the seeds, and add a scant 2 cups of the puree to the passion fruit. Mix the fruit into the cooled rosewater liquid.

5 If you have an ice-cream maker that also makes sorbets, process according to instructions. If not, pour the mixture into a flattish freezerproof dish, place in the freezer, and leave until almost frozen.

6 Remove from the freezer and break up thoroughly with a fork or puree in a food processor. Return to the freezer and repeat the process.

7 Leave in the freezer until you have the texture you require; some people like sorbets more solid than others. If yours overfreezes, transfer to the refrigerator 2 hours before serving.

fruit chocolate fondue

Here's the most romantic of desserts, as the theobromine in dark chocolate triggers feelings of love and affection. In spite of the chocolate and a very modest amount of light cream, this is a light and refreshing dessert extremely rich in healing enzymes, minerals, and vitamins and with a very high ORAC score.

1 large mango
1 small pineapple
1 cup small strawberries
2 bananas
1 small bunch red grapes
8 squares good-quality dark chocolate—preferably organic
1/2 cup light cream
2 tablespoons kirsch or Grand Marnier liqueur

1 First prepare the fruit: Cut into bite-size pieces, arrange on four plates, and refrigerate until you're ready to serve.

2 Cut or break the chocolate into small pieces and put into a fondue pot or small saucepan. Add the cream and cook over a low heat until dissolved. Don't allow it to boil.

3 Stir in the liqueur.

4 If using a fondue set, take it to the table and use the forks to dip the fruit into the chocolate. If you made the fondue in a pan, simply pour the sauce over or next to the fruit and serve immediately.

blueberry and prune muffins

It's hard to believe, but this recipe really works. In fact, you can substitute an equivalent weight of prune puree for fat in most baking recipes. Because of their natural sweetness, you can also reduce the amount of sugar, making these the healthiest muffins you've ever tasted—have two.

10 large pitted prunes
3/4 cup all-purpose white flour
3/4 cup whole-wheat flour
2 teaspoons baking powder
2 tablespoons superfine sugar
1 free-range organic egg, beaten
1/2 cup plus 2 tablespoons 2% milk
2/3 cup blueberries

1 Preheat the oven to 400°F and grease eight deep muffin cups.

2 Make the prune puree by blending the prunes in a food processor with a little water until they have the consistency of heavy cream.

3 Mix together the flours, baking powder, and sugar.

4 Mix together the egg, milk, and prune puree. Add to the flour mixture and beat thoroughly.

5 Mix in the blueberries, being careful not to break up the fruit.

6 Divide the mixture between the muffin cups, filling only to just over half their depth, and bake for 25 minutes or until a skewer inserted into the center comes out clean.

ORAC value per serving ★

papaya and couscous dessert

You've probably never eaten couscous as a dessert, as it's nearly always served as a salad, but I strongly recommend this luscious dish. You'll get lots of beta-carotene from the papaya, minerals and some vitamin C from the fruit juice, no fat, no added sugar—and it's just as good hot or cold.

2 cups unsweetened cherry juice (or cranberry or
*   unfiltered apple juice)*
3/4 cup couscous
1 large or 2 small papayas, peeled, seeded, and sliced
*   lengthwise*

1 Put the juice in a large saucepan and bring to a simmer.

2 Add the couscous gradually, allowing it to soak up the liquid. You may need to add a little more or less, depending on the quality of couscous.

3 Serve the couscous hot or cold with the fruit arranged on top.

ORAC value per serving ★★★

honeyed fruit kabobs

I was first served pineapple and cinnamon kabobs by one of London's great Indian chefs at the fabulous Chor Bazaar. This adaptation adds extra nutrients from the raspberries, mango, and papaya, and although it's a bit more complex, the increase in ORAC score is worth the effort.

1 pineapple
1 large mango, not too ripe
1 large papaya, not too ripe
2 bananas
1/2 cup honey
1/2 cup red grape juice
1/2 teaspoon cinnamon
2 teaspoons butter
1 1/2 cups raspberries

1 Prepare the pineapple, mango, papaya, and bananas and cut into evenly sized cubes.

2 Melt the honey in the grape juice in a saucepan over low heat.

3 Add the cinnamon and butter, stir well until the butter melts, and keep on a very low heat.

4 Thread the pieces of cubed fruit onto kabob skewers. Brush with the honey mixture.

5 Put under the broiler—or onto a barbecue—and cook for 3 minutes each side. Serve immediately on a bed of raspberries, with any leftover honey mixture poured on top.

ORAC value per serving ★ ★ ★

prune and chocolate terrine

Everyone needs to sin occasionally, and I could hardly deny that butter, chocolate, eggs, cream, and sugar are a bit sinful when you eat them all at once. But as you lick your lips after this amazing dish, you'll know that your indulgence has been tempered with the protective benefits of ORAC.

About 2¼ cups hot tea
1 cup prunes
5½ tablespoons unsalted butter
6 squares good-quality semisweet chocolate—preferably organic
3 free-range organic eggs, separated
1 cup heavy cream
2 tablespoons superfine brown sugar
¼ cup organic cocoa powder
1 cup large, seedless green grapes, halved

1 Pour the tea over the prunes and leave to soak for about 12 hours, then drain.

2 Melt the butter gently in a saucepan. Break the chocolate into small pieces and melt gently in the butter.

3 Beat the egg whites until stiff peaks form.

4 Beat the cream until stiff peaks form.

5 Beat the egg yolks, sugar, and cocoa together, then add the melted chocolate.

6 Add the cream and egg whites and stir in gently until smooth.

7 Line an 8-cup loaf pan neatly with parchment paper and spoon in half the mixture. Arrange half the grapes on top, cover with the prunes, and put the remaining grapes on top of the prunes.

8 Spoon in the remaining chocolate mixture.

9 Freeze until firm—about 6 hours.

10 About 2 hours before serving, remove the terrine from the freezer and from the pan and allow to soften.

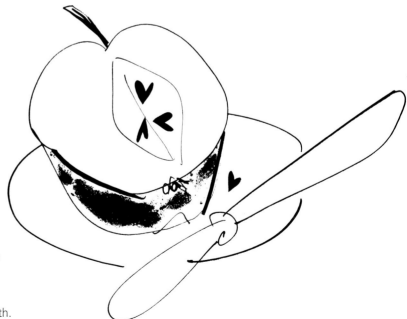

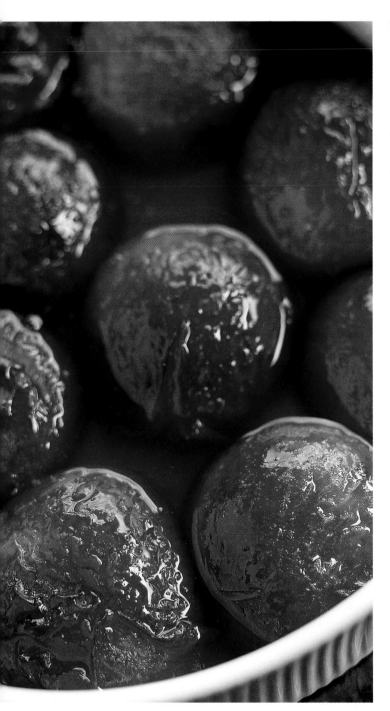

ORAC value per serving ★★⌐

plums baked in red wine and cranberry juice

This is a very simple but different dessert with a variety of health benefits. The cranberry juice helps relieve cystitis, the fresh mint makes it an excellent digestive, the red wine is good for your heart, and the plums provide fiber, vitamins, and minerals.

¹/₄ cup unsalted butter
¹/₄ cup brown sugar, blended for 30 seconds
8 plump red plums, halved and pitted
2 cups mixed red wine and cranberry juice
4 large sprigs mint, finely chopped

1 Preheat the oven to 350°F.

2 Rub the bottom of a shallow casserole dish with half the butter. Sprinkle with half the sugar and lay the plums on top, cut side down. Pour in the wine and cranberry juice and sprinkle with the mint.

3 Dot the rest of the butter on top and dust with the remaining sugar.

4 Bake for 20 minutes.

ORAC value per serving ★↗

prune soufflé

Don't be nervous about soufflés and don't worry if they don't always turn out right—I've seen great chefs take a dish of collapsed goo out of the oven. This dish really is worth a try, as the texture and flavor are remarkable, and the wafting aroma of alcoholic coffee will make your mouth water long before you take the first spoonful.

2/3 cup pitted prunes
1/4 cup chopped mixed nuts
3/4 cup fresh bread crumbs
1 tablespoon brown sugar
1/2 teaspoon allspice
1 teaspoon grated lemon rind
1 tablespoon lemon juice
1 tablespoon Tia Maria
2 free-range organic eggs, separated

1 Preheat the oven to 350°F, and lightly grease a 5-cup soufflé dish.

2 Boil the prunes in just enough water to cover for 10 minutes. Drain, reserving the liquid. Puree the prunes in a food processor until smooth.

3 Mix the nuts, bread crumbs, sugar, and allspice in a large bowl, then stir in the prune mixture. Mix in the lemon rind and lemon juice, Tia Maria, and egg yolks.

4 Stir in 5 tablespoons of the prune liquid, making up the quantity with water if necessary.

5 Whisk the egg whites until stiff and gently fold into the prune mixture. Spoon the mixture into the soufflé dish and bake for 40 minutes or until risen. Serve immediately.

ORAC value per serving ★★★★

ORAC brûlée

The ultimate healthy indulgence—go on, you deserve it! And with its enormous ORAC rating, it will do you good, too.

5 1/2 cups mixed blueberries, blackberries, strawberries,
    raspberries, and pitted cherries
1 1/4 cups heavy cream
1 cup plain organic yogurt
1/4 cup raw sugar

1 Put the fruit into one large ovenproof dish or four large (4-inch) ovenproof ramekins.

2 Beat the cream until thick, then mix in the yogurt thoroughly. Spread this mixture over the fruit, covering it completely. Sprinkle with the sugar.

3 Put under a very hot broiler until the sugar is caramelized, 3–5 minutes.

4 Allow to cool slightly before serving or refrigerate and serve cold.

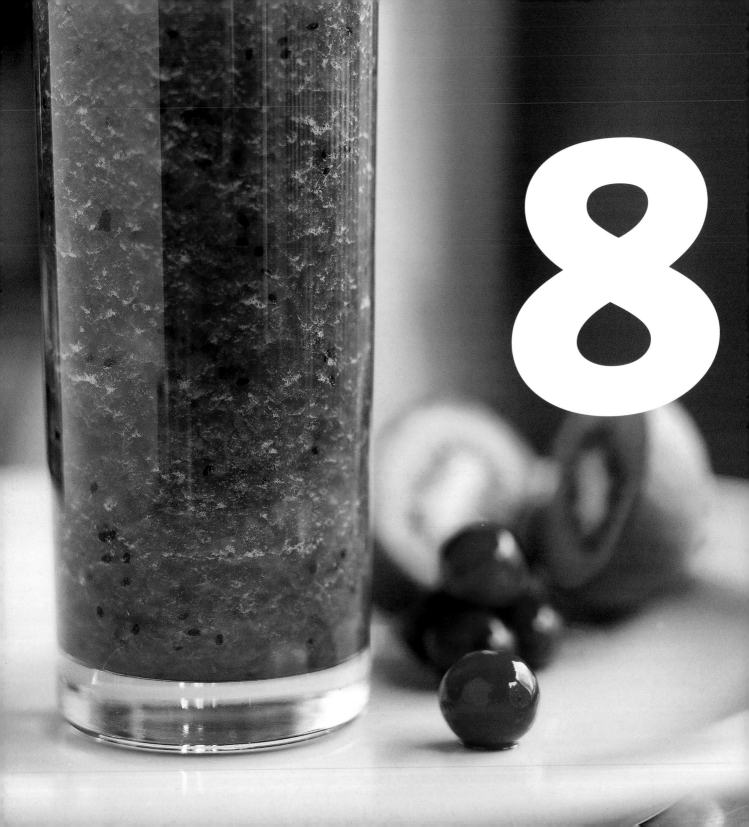

8

juices & smoothies

All recipes in this chapter make 2 large glasses

juices

In terms of health, flavor, nutrition, and ORAC scores, fresh, homemade juice comes out on top in every respect. Most kitchens today will have some kind of blender or food processor, even if it is stuck away in a cabinet. And you need one of these to make smoothies.

Unfortunately, they're no good for juices and, in my experience, juicing attachments for multipurpose machines are a waste of space and money. They're not very efficient, they're annoying, and they seldom get used. Juicing machines are now easily available and come in two types: centrifugal and masticating. If you've never juiced before, start with an inexpensive centrifugal machine. All the leading manufacturers, such as Braun and Kenwood, have good models at reasonable prices.

Centrifugal machines spin the residue into a container or filter, and in small machines this limits how much juice you can make before having to stop and clean it out. More expensive but more efficient is the Waring Professional in fashionable stainless steel, with a much larger filter—and it produces more juice. My favorite juicer of this type is the Superjuicer, which is fairly quiet, efficient, easy to clean, and has the great advantage of throwing the pulp out of the machine and into a plastic bag. This allows you to make as much juice as you want without stopping.

Masticating juicers crush the fruit and vegetables between stainless-steel rollers and are the most efficient of all. They run at lower temperatures (which protects the enzymes), extract much more of the juice, and push the pulp out the other end of the machine. They'll take frozen fruits to make instant sorbets, grind seeds and nuts—you can make your own peanut butter—and some of them will even grind flour. They are, naturally, much more expensive and bulkier, but if you're a serious juicer, invest in one of these and you have a machine that will last a lifetime. I use two of the best machines—the Champion and Green Life, both of which I have had for some time.

You'll have seen a list of the highest-ORAC foods in the general introduction. The recipes in this chapter are just suggestions—with many of my own favorites—but they're not set in stone. Use your imagination and cater to your family's tastes. Be bold and experiment, as some of the most surprising combinations end up tasting great. Juicing is the perfect way to persuade anyone—particularly children—who's not that keen on vegetables or fruits to make up the minimum of five portions a day. My own wife, who goes green at the sight of a beet, was finally persuaded to taste one of my strange mixtures and has been hooked ever since.

The recipes given here will make two large glasses, but the proportions are just a guideline and the amount of juice you get will depend on the individual ingredients—how fresh, how ripe, how juicy. But if you have, for example, only one kiwi fruit, add another apple. If there are only two pears in your fruit bowl but you've got a bag full of carrots, just keep juicing until you have enough, even though the juice might be orange rather than green. It really doesn't matter, as a glass of freshly juiced produce will be a cornucopia of vitamins, minerals, enzymes, valuable plant chemicals, and, most important, ORAC.

Another word about preparing your fruit and vegetables for juicing: It depends very much on the type of machine you're using, so look at the instructions. There's no need to peel or core apples or pears, and you don't need to remove the skin from any fruit or vegetables, even kiwis. The more robust juicers will even cope with unpeeled pineapples. If you're using organic produce, just wash it well before juicing, but if it's not organic, wash it in warm water with 1 teaspoon of liquid detergent to 4 cups of water. Scrub hard vegetables and fruits and, obviously, be more gentle with soft fruits, and make sure you rinse them well. Nonorganic carrots should be topped and tailed, and if you're juicing for children, I'd recommend peeling the carrots to be on the safe side.

Most machines will juice citrus fruits such as oranges and grapefruit if you peel them first, but thin-skinned tangerines and lemons can be used unpeeled, although this does give a slightly bitter tang to the finished juice. Anything with a very tough skin, such as avocado, passion fruit, mango, or papaya, will need to be peeled and any large central pits or seeds removed. Mango skin can cause a contact allergy—mangoes are related to poison ivy—so if you're preparing lots of them at the same time, it's sensible to wear thin rubber gloves.

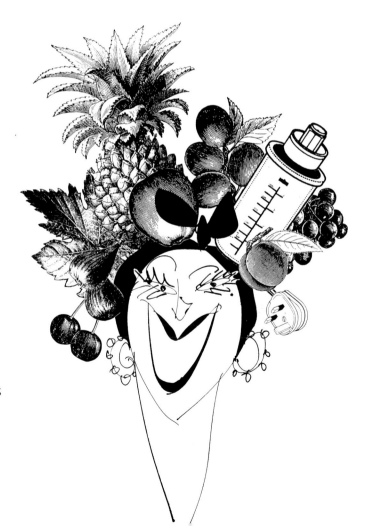

ORAC value per glass ★★★

kiwi fruit, raspberry, and blueberry

2 large kiwi fruit
3/4 cup mixed raspberries and blueberries
1 cup unfiltered organic apple juice
1 cup cranberry juice

ORAC value per glass ★★✦

carrot, apple, and kiwi fruit

4 large carrots
3 good-flavored eating apples
3 kiwi fruit

ORAC value per glass ★

carrot, sweet potato, and celery

4 large carrots
2 sweet potatoes
3 celery ribs

ORAC value per glass ★

beet, apple, and carrot

1 beet, with leaves
2 apples
3 carrots

ORAC value per glass ★★✦

cucumber, beet, and chard

1 cucumber
1 beet
3 cups Swiss chard or baby spinach

ORAC value per glass ★★

tomato, celery, radish, and red bell pepper

4 large tomatoes
3 celery ribs
12 radishes
1 red bell pepper

ORAC value per glass ★✦

pear, apple, and blueberry

3 Conference pears
2 large dessert apples
3/4 cup blueberries

ORAC value per glass ★★★

orange, carrot, spinach, and ginger

2 large oranges
1 carrot
3 cups baby spinach
1 inch fresh ginger, peeled

ORAC value per glass ★★★

strawberry, blueberry, cranberry, and red grape

1 cup strawberries
³/4 cup blueberries
¹/2 cup thawed frozen cranberries
²/3 cup seedless red grapes

ORAC value per glass ★★★★★

prune, apple, blackberry, and mango

10 pitted prunes soaked overnight in 1¹/4 cups apple juice
1 cup blackberries
1 mango

ORAC value per glass ★★★

orange, pink grapefruit, lime, and raspberry

2 oranges
1 pink grapefruit
2 limes
³/4 cup raspberries

ORAC value per glass ★★★

blueberry, cranberry, and black currant cooler

³/4 cup blueberries
¹/2 cup thawed frozen cranberries
1 cup black currants
Handful of ice cubes

ORAC value per glass ✦

traditional Bellini

3 large peaches
¹/2 bottle iced champagne

Juice the peaches. Pour into flutes and top with champagne.

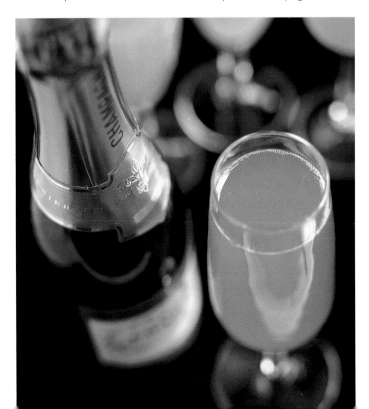

smoothies

Making smoothies couldn't be simpler. All you need is a blender or food processor, your choice of prepared fresh fruit, soft vegetables, or salad ingredients, and a milk- or soy-based liquid to bind it all together. All the ingredients are liquidized together in a matter of minutes. If you have a juicer, you can make your own juice from tougher vegetables like carrots; if not, there are several ranges of excellent commercially prepared organic vegetable juices in most supermarkets.

Smoothies are ideal if you're having problems getting enough fruit into your diet—or, more important, your children's. These creamy drinks made at home are about as far as you can get from the commercially made, chemical-ridden shakes your kids get in fast-food restaurants, and they're just as delicious. You can vary the texture and consistency to suit your or your family's preferences. Thick enough to eat with a spoon or thin enough to drink through a straw—it's entirely up to you. Add a scoop of the kids' favorite ice cream, throw in a few ice cubes while blending, or, for the adults, turn them into sophisticated "smoothtails" by adding a measure of any sweet liqueur: cherry brandy, Cointreau, crème de menthe, Galliano, or Kahlua. You could also throw in a slug of vodka, gin, Jack Daniel's, or whatever liquor appeals to you.

Smoothies provide lots of energy, loads of vitamin C, and a quarter of your daily calcium requirement; those based on yogurt also provide plenty of the good bacteria that make your digestion work more efficiently and boost your natural immunity.

As with the juices earlier in this chapter, the recipes here are just a selection of my particular favorites and ideas given to me by friends and, very often, my patients. Smoothies are a great way to experiment with flavors—and kids love to come up with something that they can call their own invention.

ORAC value per glass ★★★

strawberry, banana, and blueberry

4 large strawberries
1 small banana
3/4 cup blueberries
2 cups plain organic yogurt

ORAC value per glass ★★★★✈

soy milk, prune juice, and blueberry

1 cup soy milk
1/2 cup unsweetened prune juice
  (store bought or homemade)
3/4 cup blueberries

ORAC value per glass ★★★

avocado, papaya, yogurt, chili, and mint

2 large avocados
1 large papaya
2 cups plain organic yogurt
3 small, fresh red chilies, seeded
6 large mint leaves

ORAC value per glass ★✈

banana, strawberry, kiwi fruit, milk, and honey

1 banana
1 cup strawberries
2 kiwi fruit
2²/3 cups whole milk
2 tablespoons honey

ORAC value per glass ★✈

kiwi fruit, cherry, grape, and yogurt

3 kiwi fruit
1/2 cup fresh pitted cherries
2/3 cup seedless green grapes
2 cups plain organic yogurt

ORAC value per glass ★

passion fruit, pineapple, banana, and yogurt

6 passion fruit, pressed firmly through a strainer to get
  rid of the seeds
1 small or 1/2 large pineapple
2 bananas
2 cups plain organic yogurt

ORAC value per glass ★

pineapple, mango, banana, and coconut milk

1 small pineapple
1 mango
2 bananas
1³/4 cups canned coconut milk

ORAC value per glass ★⌐

apple, pear, plum, yogurt, and honey

3 dessert apples
2 Conference pears
6 plums
1³/4 cups plain organic yogurt
2 tablespoons honey

ORAC value per glass ⌐

beet, cucumber, yogurt, mint, and garlic

2 small, cooked beets, finely cubed
¹/2 cucumber, peeled and seeded
1³/4 cups plain organic yogurt
20 mint leaves
2 garlic cloves

ORAC value per glass ★★

banana, strawberry, and blueberry

1 small banana
1 cup strawberries
³/4 cup blueberries
2 cups plain organic yogurt

ORAC value per glass ★

pineapple, mango, and papaya with soy milk and ginger

1 pineapple
1 mango
1 papaya
2²/3 cups soy milk
1 inch peeled ginger

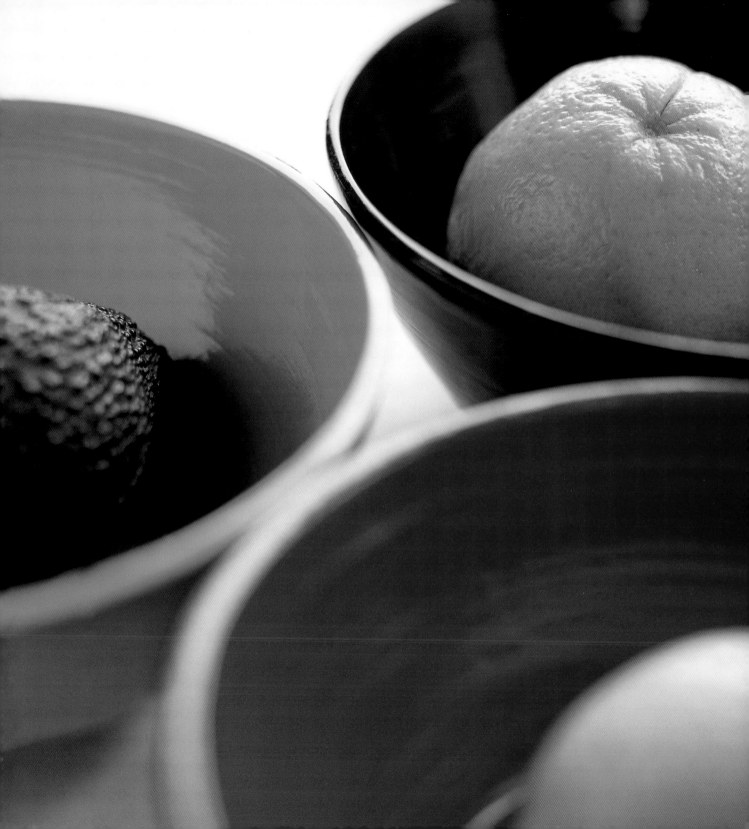

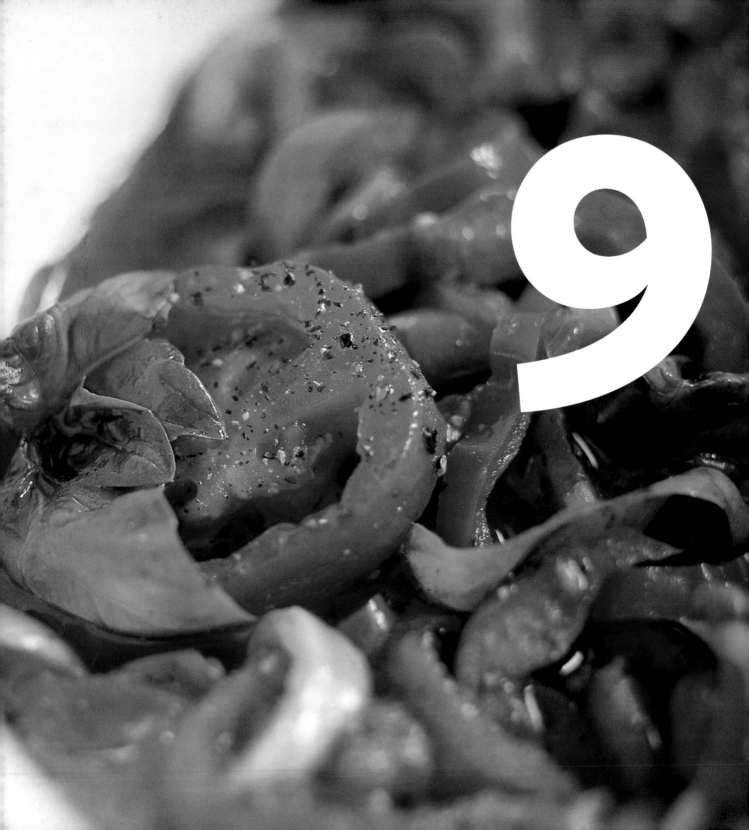

sauces,
marinades,
& compotes

All the recipes in this book have valuable ORAC scores, but using these sauces and extras will give them a valuable boost. In addition, adding them to any of your other favorite recipes, even those with low scores, will help boost their ORAC rating and increase the life-protecting value of your cooking.

savory sauces

ORAC value per average serving

fresh tomato sauce

The huge concentration of lycopene in tomato paste, combined with canned tomatoes and carrot, makes this an all-purpose savory sauce or dip.

1/4 cup olive oil
6 tablespoons tomato paste
2³/4 cups canned organic crushed tomatoes
1/2 teaspoon superfine sugar
1 carrot, shredded
Leaves of 4 large sprigs fresh basil, roughly torn
Salt and pepper

1 Heat the oil in a saucepan.

2 Stir in the tomato paste, crushed tomatoes, and sugar.

3 Add the carrot and simmer for 25 minutes, adding water if the sauce gets too thick.

4 Add the basil and simmer for an additional 5 minutes.

5 Season to taste with salt and pepper.

ORAC value per average serving ⌐

spicy tomato sauce

With loads of lycopene and the blood-positive qualities of garlic and onions, this makes a great sauce or dip.

2 tablespoons safflower oil
2 tablespoons unsalted butter
1 onion, finely chopped
2 garlic cloves, finely chopped
3 small red chilies, seeded and finely chopped
2³/4 cups canned organic crushed tomatoes

1 Heat the oil and butter in a saucepan, add the onion and garlic, and sauté them gently, stirring occasionally, until soft—about 10 minutes.

2 Add the chilies and the tomatoes to the onion mixture. Simmer gently until the mixture thickens.

ORAC value per average serving ⌐

hot tomato salsa

Extra hot and spicy, this healthy salsa is ideal as a dip or accompaniment to hot or cold dishes.

3 large tomatoes
1 red onion, very finely chopped
2 large red chilies, seeded and finely chopped
Leaves of 3 sprigs cilantro, finely chopped
¹/4 cup tomato paste

1 Peel the tomatoes by placing them in a bowl of boiling water for 2 minutes until the skins start to come away and can be slipped off easily. Chop finely.

2 Mix the tomatoes, onion, chilies, cilantro, and tomato paste together in a bowl and refrigerate for 1 hour.

ORAC value per average serving ★⌐

special applesauce

An ideal accompaniment to hot or cold dishes, and equally at home in a pancake, mixed with yogurt, rice pudding, or your breakfast cereal.

2¹/4 pounds cooking apples, cored, peeled, and sliced
¹/2 cup water
²/3 cup raisins, washed
6 whole cloves
1 tablespoon brown sugar
1¹/2 tablespoons unsalted butter

1 Place the apples in a saucepan with the water.

2 Add the raisins, cloves, and sugar and simmer the mixture gently until mushy, then remove the cloves.

3 Beat the mixture to a pulp and stir in the butter.

ORAC value per average serving

cranberry sauce

A traditional sauce with turkey, pâté, or game.

2¹/₄ cups fresh or frozen and thawed cranberries
¹/₂ cup water
3 tablespoons brown sugar

1 Wash the cranberries and pick them over carefully.

2 Beat lightly with a wooden spoon until bruised.

3 Simmer in the water and sugar until tender.

4 Push through a strainer to remove the skins and seeds.

ORAC value per average serving

gooseberry sauce

This simple and delicious sauce is equally at home on hot or cold, sweet or savory dishes—and it makes a fabulous topping for ice cream. The highest ORAC value is obtained by using sweet, red dessert gooseberries.

2¹/₄ cups ripe gooseberries, washed and picked over
2¹/₂ cups water or any wine you may have left over
3–4 tablespoons brown sugar
A generous pat of unsalted butter
2 tablespoons Calvados (optional)

1 Place the gooseberries in a saucepan with the water or wine and simmer until soft.

2 Push through a strainer to remove the skins. Return to the pan and add the sugar to taste, then the butter.

3 Reheat and stir in the Calvados.

ORAC value per average serving

horseradish sauce

Rich in highly protective sulfur compounds, horseradish is the perfect accompaniment to hot or cold roast beef and smoked fish. It's really worth growing your own or buying fresh roots when they're available. Grated and frozen, it will keep all its flavor and health properties, and although used only as a condiment, one tablespoon is a good addition to your daily ORAC consumption.

1 cup heavy or whipping cream
6 tablespoons grated horseradish—if you grow it or can find some growing wild and do it yourself, all the better
3 tablespoons white wine vinegar or cider vinegar
Salt and pepper

1 Beat the cream to thicken it.

2 Stir in the horseradish and vinegar.

3 Season to taste with salt and pepper.

ORAC value per average serving

horseradish and beet sauce

This traditional eastern European recipe is perfect with cold meats and strongly flavored fish. The combination of high-value beets with horseradish makes it even more protective.

2 large cooked (not pickled) beets, finely grated
1/2 cup grated horseradish—buy it prepared or grate the raw root yourself
About 2 tablespoons brown sugar, blended for 30 seconds
Red wine vinegar

1 Place the beets in a bowl, add the horseradish, and mix well.

2 Stir in the sugar, tasting—carefully, as it will be very hot on its own—until the sweetness suits your palate.

3 Gradually beat in just enough vinegar to bind the sauce.

ORAC value per average serving ★

orange sauce

This easy-to-make and delicately sweet-and-sour sauce is ideal with duck, goose, venison, or smoked sausage. It's rich in vitamin C and has good ORAC value, too.

3 tablespoons grated orange rind
2/3 cup red currant jelly
3 tablespoons brown sugar
1 1/2 cups freshly squeezed orange juice
2 tablespoons lemon juice
2 pinches paprika
3 tablespoons port or brandy

1 Beat the orange rind, red currant jelly, and sugar in a blender.

2 Pour the mixture into a saucepan, add the orange and lemon juices, paprika, and port or brandy, and heat through, adding more paprika for a spicier taste.

ORAC value per average serving

Cumberland sauce

This is a traditional sauce, usually served with coarse terrines and cold potpies, like game, pork, or veal and ham. I think it also goes well with strong cheeses, such as a really mature organic farmhouse cheddar.

2 tablespoons grated orange rind
4 teaspoons grated lemon rind
1 cup freshly squeezed orange juice
1/4 cup lemon juice
2 tablespoons mild mustard
1 tablespoon superfine sugar
1/2 cup red currant jelly
1/2 teaspoon cayenne pepper
1/4 cup red wine
2 tablespoons port

1 Simmer the grated orange and lemon rinds in water until softened—about 4 minutes. Drain.

2 Put the orange and lemon juices in another pan. Add the grated rinds, mustard, sugar, red currant jelly, cayenne pepper, and wine. Simmer very gently for about 5 minutes, adding more wine if the mixture gets too thick.

3 Stir in the port.

sweet sauces

ORAC value per average serving ★

raspberry sauce

Nothing quite matches the taste of raspberries, and when combined with the health-giving benefits of probiotic bacteria in yogurt, the result is a delicious, immune-boosting, high-ORAC sauce.

2¹/₄ cups raspberries, washed and hulled—fresh are obviously best, frozen will do, but canned most certainly won't
¹/₄ cup kirsch or any raspberry liqueur
Confectioners' sugar
¹/₂ cup plain organic yogurt (optional)

1 Puree the raspberries with the liqueur in a blender or mash the two together thoroughly with a fork. Push through a fine strainer to remove the seeds.

2 If you like a very tart sauce, omit the sugar. Otherwise sweeten the sauce to taste.

3 If you want to make a slightly creamy sauce, stir in the yogurt.

ORAC value per average serving

yogurt sauce

Good enough to eat on its own, but wonderful served with hot or cold desserts, this sauce has good bacteria, vitamin C, and all the digestive benefits of mint.

1 heaping cup black currants, washed and hulled
2 teaspoons grated lemon rind
2 tablespoons honey
¹/₂ teaspoon cinnamon
1 large sprig mint, finely chopped
1 cup plain organic yogurt

1 Place the black currants in a saucepan with water to cover and simmer gently for 5–10 minutes, until just tender. Drain and push the berries through a fine strainer to remove the seeds. Leave the puree to cool completely.

2 Mix the lemon rind, honey, cinnamon, and mint into the yogurt.

3 When the black currant puree has cooled, stir it thoroughly into the yogurt mixture.

ORAC value per average serving ★★

three-fruit sauce

With the lemon juice taking the edge off the sweetness, this sauce is best served warm with hot or cold desserts. It's especially wonderful poured over vanilla ice cream or used on hot waffles or pancakes. Not surprisingly, it turns any dessert into an ORAC feast.

2/3 cup dried apricots
1/2 cup pitted prunes
1 cup fresh or frozen cranberries
6 tablespoons lemon juice

1 Put the dried fruit and the cranberries into a large saucepan and just cover with boiling water. Bring back to a boil, cover, and simmer until tender, checking regularly that the mixture isn't drying out.

2 Transfer the fruit with about 1/2 cup of the water to a blender and puree. (Depending on the size of your blender, you may have to do this in batches.) Reserve the remainder of the cooking water.

3 Return the puree to a dry saucepan, adding more of the cooking water if it seems too thick. Heat through and stir in the lemon juice.

ORAC value per average serving ★★★

blueberry sauce

Of all grapes, the Concord has the highest ORAC value. Mixed here with another top-ranking antioxidant food, blueberries, it provides enormous health benefits that more than make up for the small amount of sugar—whatever "naughty" dessert you decide to pour this over. It's equally good hot or cold on ice cream, apple pie, or rice pudding.

1 2/3 cups blueberries
1 cup Concord grape juice
1 tablespoon organic raw sugar
2 pinches nutmeg

Just blend all the ingredients together.

marinades

ORAC value per average serving ↱

peanut marinade and sauce

Some of the marinade will be absorbed by the food soaking in it. To get the full ORAC value, add the rest of the marinade during cooking. If using meat or fish, cook at a sufficiently high temperature to boil the added marinade and kill any bacteria that may have seeped from these foods.

1/2 cup basic stock (see page 30)
Heaping 1/4 cup smooth peanut butter
2 tablespoons soy sauce
3 garlic cloves
3 tablespoons rice vinegar or white wine vinegar
2 teaspoons brown sugar
Leaves of 2 large sprigs cilantro, roughly chopped
Leaves of 2 large sprigs Italian parsley, roughly chopped
1/2 teaspoon cayenne pepper

1 Bring the stock gently to a boil.

2 Place in a blender with the peanut butter, soy sauce, and garlic and blend until smooth.

3 Add the vinegar and sugar and blend again for 10 seconds.

4 Put the mixture into the rinsed-out saucepan. Add the herbs and the cayenne pepper and heat through.

ORAC value per average serving ↱

Mandarin's marinade

This hot recipe can be used as a marinade for meat, fish, and poultry, and is equally valuable as a hot pouring sauce. You can keep it covered in the refrigerator for three or four days. This unmistakably Asian mixture isn't an exceptionally high-ORAC recipe, but it has the bonus of being a great circulatory booster.

4 inches fresh ginger, peeled and finely grated
1/2 cup freshly squeezed orange juice
11/4 cups basic stock (see page 30) or stock made with a
  low-salt stock cube, preferably organic
6 tablespoons hoisin sauce
3 tablespoons light soy sauce
6 tablespoons rice vinegar
3 tablespoons extra-virgin olive oil
3 tablespoons sesame seed oil
5 teaspoons mild mustard

Put all the ingredients in a blender and blend until smooth.

ORAC value per average serving ⤻

basic meat marinade

As well as imparting flavor and ORAC value, these marinades actually start the cooking process and help tenderize meat and poultry. Both mint and tarragon are excellent digestive herbs and provide extra ORAC.

3 garlic cloves, very finely chopped
1 sprig rosemary, finely chopped
A few sprigs thyme, finely chopped
A few sprigs marjoram, finely chopped
1 cup red wine
1 cup extra-virgin olive oil

1 Mix the garlic and herbs into the wine and oil.

2 Baste the meat in the mixture and leave in the refrigerator for at least 2 hours.

3 Add the meat and marinade to casseroles or strain off the marinade; broil, roast, or barbecue the meat; and use the marinade as a baste or in a sauce or gravy.

For lamb: *Add 2 large stems mint.*
For poultry: *Add 4 stems tarragon.*

ORAC value per average serving ⤻

marinade for fish

Marinating fish helps bring out the wonderful flavors that are unique to each variety, and, in spite of the mixture of herbs, the marinades won't dominate the taste of your finished dish. The combination of herbs, capers, and lemon produces the ORAC score in this marinade.

1 teaspoon capers, drained
Milk
1 lemon
1 cup white wine
1 cup virgin olive oil
6 sprigs dill
3 sprigs chervil
2 sprigs parsley

1 Place the capers in enough milk to cover them and soak for 10 minutes—this removes any excessive sharpness. Drain and squash lightly. Finely grate the rind from the lemon and cut the fruit into slices.

2 Mix the wine and olive oil in a bowl. Add the capers and lemon rind and stir thoroughly. Stir in the whole sprigs of dill, chervil, and parsley.

3 Pour the marinade over the fish, top with the lemon slices, and leave in the refrigerator for 1 hour.

4 If you're broiling the fish or putting it on a barbecue, drain from the marinade, put on or under the heat, and use the juices as a baste. If you're baking, roasting, or making a casserole, use as much of the marinade as you like for flavor in the stock, in fish cooked in pockets of foil, or boiled down to make a sauce.

compotes

All these compotes have high ORAC scores and can make a considerable difference to your daily ORAC intake. It's nice to know that these delicious sweet additions to your favorite dishes have such wonderful health benefits.

ORAC value per average serving

dried fruit compote

This is perfect with cold meats, poultry, and strong cheeses.

1¹/₂ cups mixed pitted prunes, dried apricots, and golden raisins
2 teaspoons finely grated lemon rind
2 tablespoons lemon juice
1¹/₄ cups sweet white wine
3 cinnamon sticks

1 Put the dried fruit, lemon rind, and lemon juice into a large saucepan and cover with the wine.

2 Add the cinnamon sticks and simmer gently until the fruit is tender.

3 Remove the cinnamon sticks before serving.

ORAC value per average serving

fresh berry compote

This compote is wonderful with pâté, potpies, goose, venison, ham, and—best of all—cold turkey the day after Thanksgiving or Christmas, when you need all the ORAC you can get to make up for all the festive indulgences.

4³/₄ cups mixed fresh or frozen and thawed blackberries, raspberries, and red currants
¹/₄ cup organic honey

1 Wash and pick over the fruit. Put it into a saucepan and add just enough water to cover.

2 Add the honey. Simmer, stirring gently, for 2 minutes to melt the honey, then boil until most of the liquid has evaporated.

ORAC value per average serving ★

rhubarb, ginger, and gooseberry compote

This is actually good enough to eat on its own. But it's also perfect with hot or cold oily fish and smoked fish; stirred into yogurt; poured, hot or cold, over your favorite ice cream; or mixed into muesli for breakfast. For a real treat, serve with hot, homemade apple pie.

1 cup sliced rhubarb, tough fibers removed, stems cut into
  $1/2$ inch slices
$1/2$ cup gooseberries, stems removed
$1^1/4$ inches ginger, peeled and very finely grated
2 tablespoons honey
$2^1/4$ cups unsweetened elderflower cordial, diluted
  if necessary

Put the fruit, ginger, and honey into a saucepan with just enough elderflower cordial to cover. Simmer until the fruit is tender, adding more cordial if the compote becomes too dry.

ORAC value per average serving ★★★↗

warm cinnamon compote

With all its dried fruits, this delicious mixture is exceptionally high in ORAC values. It also has the added digestive bonus of the spices and a high fiber content.

1 medium cinnamon stick
1 inch peeled and finely grated ginger
2 thin slices lemon
$1/2$ cup each dried cranberries, blueberries, cherries, baby figs,
  and muscatel raisins

1 Put all the ingredients into a large bowl and cover with boiling water.

2 Soak for 1 hour at room temperature.

3 Remove the lemon slices and serve alone or with yogurt sauce (see page 126).

salad dressings

ORAC value per average serving

standard French dressing

A good salad is a true delight. The secret is in the preparation and the dressing. Wash all salad ingredients well—even those in the plastic bags that say "washed and ready to use"—and dry thoroughly. A salad spinner is the best and cheapest kitchen gadget you'll ever buy. Even the best dressing won't coat the surface of wet leaves and you end up with a soggy mess. This dressing will go with any type of salad.

6 tablespoons extra-virgin olive oil
1/4 cup herb vinegar—make your own by putting a mixture
 of sprigs of rosemary, chervil, parsley, and tarragon into
 a bottle and leaving for a least a week, or buy commercially
 produced herb vinegar
2 teaspoons mild mustard
1 teaspoon sea salt

3 generous twists freshly ground black pepper
3 tablespoons chopped mixed fresh soft herb leaves—Italian
 parsley, tarragon, marjoram, chervil, and oregano

1 Place all the ingredients except the fresh herbs in a bowl and blend with a whisk until thickened.

2 Stir in the fresh herbs.

This dressing will keep in an airtight jar for at least a week, but don't put it in the refrigerator, as it will separate.

ORAC value per average serving ★

creamy yogurt dressing

This cool, green dressing goes well with cold new potatoes, a mixed green salad, or cold fresh salmon.

3 tablespoons olive oil
1 cup plain organic yogurt
1/2 cucumber, peeled, seeded, and finely chopped
1 large green bell pepper, seeded and finely diced
1 sweet white Spanish onion, finely chopped
2 garlic cloves, finely chopped

1 Mix the yogurt and olive oil together.

2 Put all the ingredients into a blender and blend for 1 minute.

ORAC value per average serving ⌐

spicy dressing for fish salads

This refreshing dressing is perfect with any salad made with canned, fresh, or smoked tuna, or flaked steamed cod, salmon, trout, or mackerel. It's also superb on seafood salads with shrimp, crab, lobster, squid, or mussels.

1/2 cup olive oil
1/2 cup walnut oil
2 small red chilies, seeded and finely chopped
3 large scallions, trimmed and finely sliced
1 garlic clove, chopped
1 inch fresh ginger, peeled and grated

Mix all the ingredients together and leave in the refrigerator for 1 hour to allow the flavors to combine.

ORAC value per average serving ⌐

Thai dressing

Healthy eating is as much about enjoyment as it is about nutrition. Although this dressing doesn't have a particularly high ORAC score, it's reasonably high in antioxidants and extremely high in heart-protective monounsaturated oils, vitamin E, and essential trace minerals—and it tastes great on pan-fried or barbecued shrimp or chicken.

2 tablespoons oyster sauce
2 tablespoons lemon juice
2 teaspoons honey
4 large scallions, finely chopped
1/2 teaspoon paprika
1 tablespoon dry-fried sesame seeds
1/4 cup sesame oil
2 tablespoons tahini

Put all the ingredients into a blender and blend until smooth, adding more oil if necessary.

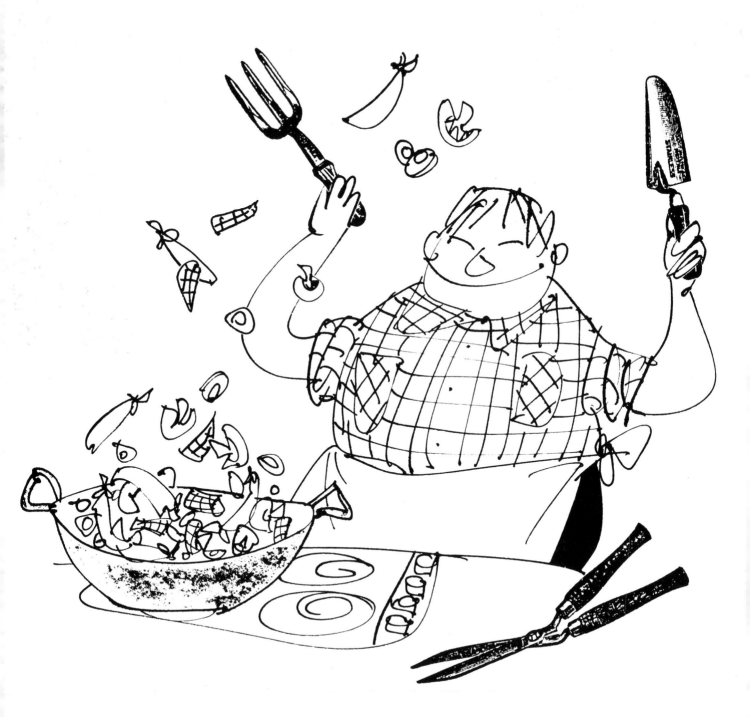

seven days of ORACle eating

If you really want to do everything you can to help your food ensure your continuing good health, there are 150 ideas in this book. It would be easy to keep your ORAC rating extremely high by eating only, say, the top five foods in the ORAC table. However, confining your food intake to prunes, raisins, blueberries, blackberries, and garlic wouldn't just be extremely dull, but you'd be missing out dangerously on a whole range of nutrients that the body needs to keep it running efficiently.

Food should be about enjoyment as much as anything else, and if you can make small changes to your diet, you can enjoy the fun as well as the health benefits. Here's a week of ORAC eating chosen to maximize your consumption of these vital foods without sacrificing the wide range of flavors and textures, which would be anathema to anyone who loves food. And remember, the ORAC values here don't take into account any additional vegetables or salads you serve with these dishes.

		page	*ORAC value*

day 1

Breakfast:	Oatmeal with prunes and raisins	22	6¹/₂
	Carrot, apple, and kiwi juice	114	2¹/₂
Lunch:	Vegetable risotto	59	2¹/₂
	Mediterranean mix	55	3
Dinner:	Steamed fish in foil	95	2¹/₂
	Plums baked in wine and cranberry juice	108	1¹/₂
	Total		**18¹/₂ stars**

day 2

Breakfast:	Fruity appetizer with beans and tomatoes	22	3
Lunch:	Tomato, mozzarella, and avocado salad	73	4
	Tea bread with raisins and prunes	102	4¹/₂
Dinner:	Cabbage and beet soup	43	4
	Stir-fried vegetables with shrimp	96	3¹/₂
	Total		**19 stars**

	page	*ORAC value*

day 3

		page	ORAC value
Breakfast:	Avocado with sliced tomato	23	2¹/₂
	Orange, pink grapefruit, lime, and raspberry juice	115	3
Lunch:	Stuffed red peppers	62	3
	Strawberry, banana, and blueberry smoothie	117	3
Dinner:	Braised duck with prunes	90	7
	Watercress, Belgian endive, and alfalfa salad	52	4
	Total		**22¹/₂ stars**

day 4

		page	ORAC value
Breakfast:	Fruit-filled melon shells	25	4
Lunch:	Shrimp couscous with raisins	66	2¹/₂
	Blueberry and prune muffins	105	5
Dinner:	Mango chicken	79	2¹/₂
	Tabbouleh with a difference	51	1¹/₂
	Fruity rice pudding	100	5
	Total		**20¹/₂ stars**

		page	*ORAC value*

day 5

		page	ORAC value
Breakfast:	Swiss muesli with blueberries	24	5
	Strawberry, blueberry, cranberry, and grape juice	115	3
Lunch:	Broccoli, cauliflower, and cheese	59	3
	Beet, pink grapefruit, and red onion salad	46	2
Dinner:	Curried bean and root vegetable stew	89	3
	Chilled cherry soup	39	4
		Total	**20 stars**

day 6

		page	ORAC value
Breakfast:	Compote of dried fruits with yogurt and flaxseeds	27	6
Lunch:	Tuna fishcakes	68	2
	Wild and red rice on radicchio	48	1$\frac{1}{2}$
Dinner:	Cheat's gazpacho	34	2$\frac{1}{2}$
	Vegetarian nutty bake	83	3$\frac{1}{2}$
	Prune and chocolate terrine	107	3$\frac{1}{2}$
		Total	**19 stars**

		page	*ORAC value*

day 7

Breakfast:	Deviled prunes with spicy tomato sauce	25	6$\frac{1}{2}$
	Kiwi, raspberry, and blueberry juice	114	3
Lunch:	Traditional salade niçoise	49	1
	Blueberry, cranberry, and black currant cooler	115	3
Dinner:	Cream of broccoli and Brussels sprouts soup	40	2
	ORAC brûlée	109	4
	Total		**19$\frac{1}{2}$ stars**

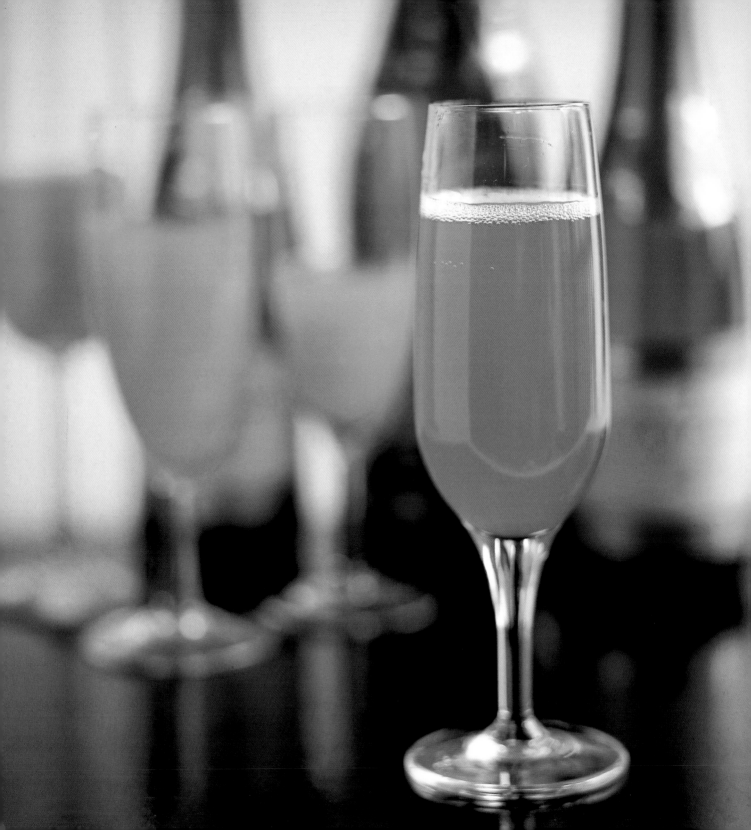

index

acknowledgments

I'd like to dedicate this book to my wife, Sally, as without her support during my long and tedious recovery from an accident, it would never have been written. She also developed and tested all the recipes, as well as cooking and styling the food for the photographs.

I'd also like to thank Ray Main and his assistant, Leigh, for taking such fabulous pictures, and Marie-Hélène Jeeves for her cartoons. Needless to say, without the encouragement of Kyle Cathie and her staff, and the untiring efforts of my secretary, Janet, *The ORACle Diet* would not exist.

Finally, a special thank-you to one of the unsung heroes of healthy eating. Sham Grimshaw runs one of the best wholesale companies at New Covent Garden Market and supplies some of the best chefs and grandest dining rooms in London. I'm happy to say that he has also supplied me with the freshest, healthiest, and most delicious selection of every imaginable type of fruit, vegetable, herb, and salad.

Laurel Glen Publishing
An imprint of the Advantage Publishers Group
5880 Oberlin Drive, San Diego, CA 92121-4794
www.laurelglenbooks.com

This edition published in 2003
First published in Great Britain in 2002 by Kyle Cathie Limited

Text © Michael van Straten 2002
Layout © Kyle Cathie Limited 2002
Drawings © Marie-Hélène Jeeves 2002
Photographs © Ray Main 2002

Copyright under International, Pan American, and Universal Copyright Conventions. All rights reserved. No part of this book may be reproduced or transmitted in any form or by any means, electronic or mechanical, including photocopying, recording, or by any information storage-and-retrieval system, without written permission from the copyright holder. Brief passages (not to exceed 1,000 words) may be quoted for reviews.

All notations of errors or omissions should be addressed to Laurel Glen Publishing, Editorial Department, at the above address. All other correspondence (author inquiries, permissions and rights) concerning the content of this book should be addressed to Kyle Cathie Ltd, 122 Arlington Road, London NW1 7HP, U.K., or generalenquiries@kyle-cathie.com.

ISBN 1-59223-186-1
Library of Congress Cataloging-in-Publication Data available upon request.

Edited by Barbara Horn
Designed by Geoff Hayes
Production by Lorraine Baird and Sha Huxtable

Color separations by Colourscan
Printed and bound in Singapore
1 2 3 4 5   08 07 06 05 04